Mainstreaming Equality in the European Union

Education, Training and Labour Market Policies

Teresa Rees

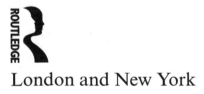

London and New York

First published 1998
by Routledge
11 New Fetter Lane, London EC4P 4EE

Simultaneously published in the USA and Canada
by Routledge
29 West 35th Street, New York, NY 10001

Typeset in Times by Routledge
Printed and bound in Great Britain by Creative Print and Design
(Wales), Ebbw Vale

British Library Cataloguing in Publication Data
A catalogue record for this book is available from the British Library

Library of Congress Cataloguing-in-Publication Data
Rees, Teresa L.
Mainstreaming equality in the European union / Teresa Rees.
Includes bibliographical references and index.
1. Women–Employment–European Union Countries. 2. Manpower
policy–European Union countries. 3.Occupational training for
women–European Union countries. 4. Sex discrimination in
employment–European Union countries. 5. Labor market–European
Union countries.
HD6134.5.R44   1988
                                        331.4'094–dc21 97–17427
                                                                CIP

ISBN 0–415–11533–7 (hbk)
ISBN 0–415–11534–5 (pbk)

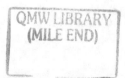

Contents

List of tables

Preface

For the past six years, I have been in the somewhat daunting position of being hired as an expert advisor to the European Commission (EC) on equal opportunities and training policy. If at times I felt that the value of what I was learning was considerably greater than that which I was imparting, this is probably because it was so. Fortunately, rather obvious questions posed by the outsider can sometimes sound disarmingly insightful. Despite such concerns I have very much appreciated the opportunity afforded me by the Commission to bring some insights from feminist theory to bear on the tricky business of trying to do something about equal opportunities in the labour force at a European level. Given my conviction that vocational education and training systems for the most part underpin patterns of gender segregation in the labour force, and reinforce features of work organisation and culture that disadvantage women, the opportunity to be involved in the development of policies and programmes seeking to deliver equal opportunities and skill enhancement to women was too attractive to resist.

As time went on, and I heard myself referring to companies as 'enterprises' and to trade unions and employers' associations as 'social partners', and when friends and colleagues began to pick my brains on acronyms and abbreviations, when French and German phrases and even Eurospeak words such as subsidiarity, animation and synergy began sporadically and spontaneously to pepper my speech, I realised I had gone over to the other side. I had become one of those people who knows something of the maze which is the European Union (EU). The EC, with its Directives and Directorate-Generals, its programmes, policies and projects, had become, to an extent at least, familiar territory. It was this realisation that prompted me to write this book. It is an attempt to share what I have learned, researched and analysed with those concerned with and about gender segregation in education, training and the labour force in the EU.

The issue of gender segregation has been the subject of considerable academic and policy attention. This book focuses on the attempts made at the European level to incorporate equal opportunities into education and training policies. It examines in particular the evolution of approaches towards equal opportunities in policies and programmes. It analyses these shifts in terms of a conceptual framework which differentiates between equal treatment, positive action and discrimination, and, finally, the idea of 'feminising the mainstream' or 'mainstreaming equality'. The concept of mainstreaming is as yet underdeveloped in the literature, but I judge it to have some potential to reduce significantly the impact of gender on educational, training and occupational lifechances.

The book has been written in what I hope is a jargon-free style to be accessible not just to academics and students interested in this area but to those grappling with equal opportunities policies in education and training policy or practice. It draws upon experiences of transnational women's training projects to illustrate the need to adopt a radical overhaul of mainstream training provision, if women's skills are to be developed significantly.

I owe an enormous debt of gratitude to a considerable number of people who have contributed directly or indirectly to the production of this book. First of all, I would like to thank those individuals within the EC who gave me the opportunity to work with them in developing ideas and policies. Above all I am grateful to Frances Smith of DGXXII who has been my liaison person in the Commission throughout the last six years. She has provided a very positive response to ideas which ranged from the practical to the hopelessly idealistic, not to say zany. I have had the pleasure (tinged with fear) of seeing many of my suggestions taken up and turned into action through her initiative, commitment and energy. She has pursued the equality agenda vigorously and imaginatively and, in my view, has made a significant impact on the extent to which women are likely to benefit from EC programmes in the future. She has also provided many home comforts for a Brit abroad.

Hywel Ceri Jones, Deputy Director of the EC's Directorate General Employment and Social Affairs (DGV), whose commitment to equal opportunities is demonstrated in his thinking and his actions, commissioned me to undertake some of the work upon which this book draws when he was the Director of the Task Force Human Resources Education, Training and Youth (now DGXXII). His successor, Tom O'Dwyer, kindly continued that commitment and support.

I received tremendous cooperation and support from Commission staff, both in DGXXII, DGV and the Technical Assistance Offices (TAOs) of the community action programmes, for which I am most grateful. Colleagues in the Centre for Research on European Women (CREW), the University Enterprise Training Partnerships (UETPs), particularly Women Into Technology (WITEC), and elsewhere have provided most valuable assistance (these acronyms will, hopefully, slide easily from your tongue, too, by the time you reach the end of the book).

Sara Delamont and Caroline Joll of the University of Wales Cardiff provided me with detailed and thoughtful feedback on an earlier draft, for which I am most grateful. Other friends and colleagues have been enormously important in the development of my ideas about mainstreaming and women and training. They include Catherine Eva of the Welsh Development Agency, Val Feld from the Equal Opportunities Commission in Wales, Glenys Kinnock, MEP, Jane Hutt from Chwarae Teg (Welsh for 'Fair Play'), Janet Smith, an independent consultant, and Neil Wooding, equality advisor for the NHS in Wales. Transnational partnerships have provided a verdant learning experience. I learnt from Pat Brand from Dublin that it was important to trust foreigners' ways of seeing and doing. Frédérique Deroure taught me the difference between French and Anglo-Saxon logic. Discussions with Mario Bucci showed me that good ideas can travel. Jenny Capstick provided enormous assistance in making the manuscript presentable and the references coherent. Heather Gibson of Routledge proved patient while persistent, which ensured the book was complete if not perfect.

Family and friends have provided considerable support during the years of work upon which this book draws. I should like especially to thank Gareth, Ieuan and Dyfrig Rees, and friends from Cardiff and Bristol, particularly Paul Atkinson, Martin Boddy, Gill Boden, Gary Bridge, Sara Delamont, Kevin Doogan, Caroline Joll, Anne Murcott and Chris Weedon, all of whom provided support and encouragement when the project (and indeed at times, life itself) appeared to be too complex and difficult to fathom.

Abbreviations and acronyms

ADAPT	Community Initiative for the Adaptation of Workers to Industrial Change
ADAPT-BIS	Community Initiative for the Adaptation of Workers to Industrial Change: Building an Information Society
APL	Accreditation of Prior Learning
ARION	Actleprogramma: Reizen met een Instructief Paracter voor Onderwijss (EC Programme for study visits for educationalists)
ATHENA	FORCE project on women and skill shortages
AXIA	Transnational project on women employees' training needs
BIBB	Bundesinstitut für Berufsbildung (Centre for the development of vocational training) (Germany)
BTEC	Business and Technology and Education Council
CEC	Commission of the European Communities
CEDEFOP	European Centre for the Development of Vocational Training
CEEP	European Centre of Enterprises with Public Participation
CIS	Commonwealth of Independent States

COMETT	Community action programme for Education and Training for Technology
COPEC	EC's Equal Opportunities Committee
CoR	Committee of the Regions
CREW	Centre for Research on European Women
CSF	Community Support Frameworks
DE	Department of Employment
DfEE	Department for Education and Employment (UK)
DG	Directorate-General
EAGGF	European Agricultural Guidance and Guarantee Fund
EC	European Commission
ECILWC	EC Centre for the Improvement of Living and Working Conditions
ECJ	European Court of Justice
ECOSOC	Economic and Social Committee
EEA	European Economic Area
EEC	European Economic Community
EFTA	European Free Trade Association
EMPLOYMENT	Community Initiative for Employment and Development of Human Resources
ENOW	European Network of Women
ENTP	European Network of Training Partnerships
EO	Equal opportunities
EOC	Equal Opportunities Commission (GB)
EOC NI	Equal Opportunities Commission (Northern Ireland)
ERASMUS	European Action Scheme for the Mobility of University Students
ERDF	European Regional Development Fund
ERGO	Community action programme for the long-term unemployed
ESF	European Social Fund
ETUC	European Trade Union Confederation
EU	European Union
EUROPS	European Office for Programme Support for the Community Initiatives ADAPT and EMPLOYMENT

Eurostat	Statistical Office of the European Communities
EUROTECNET	Network of Demonstration Projects on Vocational Training and New Information Technologies
EWL	European Women's Lobby
FORCE	Development of Continuing Training in Firms
FT	Foundation Targets (NVQs)
GB	Great Britain
GCE	General Certificate of Education (UK)
GCSE	General Certificate of Secondary Education (UK)
GDP	Gross Domestic Product
GNVQs	General National Vocational Qualifications (UK)
GSOH	Good sense of humour
HELIOS	Action programme for the Vocational and Social Integration of Handicapped Persons
HORIZON	Initiative for the Handicapped and Disadvantaged Persons Inter-University Cooperation Programme (strand in DGV EMPLOYMENT Initiative)
ICP	Inter-University Cooperation Programme
IGC	Intergovernmental Conference
IIP	Investors in People
ILO	International Labour Organization
IMG	Individual Mobility Grants (TEMPUS)
INTEGRA	Strand in DGV EMPLOYMENT Initiative targeted at the disadvantaged
IRDAC	Industrial Research and Development Advisory Committee of the Commission of the European Communities
IRIS	European Network of vocational training projects for women

ISFOL	Institute for the development of vocational training for workers (Italy)
JEPs	Joint European Projects (TEMPUS)
JSA	Job Seekers' Allowance (UK)
LECs	Local Enterprise Companies (Scotland)
LEI	Local Employment Initiatives
LEONARDO DA VINCI	Community Initiative on Vocational Training
LFS	Labour Force Survey
LINGUA	Action Programme on Modern Language Teaching
LTs	Lifetime Targets (NVQs)
MEP	Member of European Parliament
NACETT	National Advisory Council for Education and Training Targets
NCUs	National Coordination Units
NGAA	National Grant Awarding Authority
NITS	New information technologies
NOW	New Opportunities for Women (strand in DGV EMPLOYMENT Initiative)
NS	Non-smoker
NTETS	National Targets for Education and Training (England and Wales)
NVQs	National Vocational Qualifications (UK)
OECD	Organisation for Economic Co-operation and Development
OPs	Operational Programmes
PA	Positive action
PD	Positive discrimination
PETRA	Partnership in Education and Training for Young People
PHARE	Pologne Hongrie Aide à la Reconstruction Economique (Assistance for the Economic Reconstruction of Poland and Hungary)
RACINE	Network for support and utilisation of European innovations (France)
RSA	Royal Society of Arts
SMEs	Small and medium size enterprises

SOCRATES	Community Initiative on Education
TACIS	Technical Assistance to the CIS and Georgia
TAOs	Technical Assistance Offices
TECs	Training and Enterprise Councils (England and Wales)
TEMPUS	Trans-European Mobility Programme for University Students
TFHR	Task Force Human Resources, Education, Training and Youth (now DGXXII)
UETPs	University Enterprise Training Partnerships (COMETT Programme)
UK	United Kingdom
UNICE	Union of Industrial and Employers' Confederations of Europe
US	United States of America
VET	Vocational education and training
WITEC	Women into Technology
YIP	Youth Initiative Projects (PETRA)
YOUTHSTART	Promoting Access to Work and Continuing Training of Young People (Strand in DGV EMPLOYMENT Initiative)

Chapter 1

Introduction

The principle of equal treatment for men and women was enshrined in the 1957 Treaty of Rome which set up the European Economic Community (EEC), long before the issue had become one of significance in many of its constituent Member States.[1] However, in the late 1990s, despite equality legislation, a greater awareness of the social justice argument for equal opportunities and the 'business case' being made by both sides of industry (CEC and Social Dialogue 1993), gender segregation remains one of the most entrenched characteristics of the labour force in the European Union (EU). While patterns of segregation may shift and change with the restructuring of the labour market, reflecting the demise of some occupations and sectors and the emergence of others, nevertheless men and women remain fixed in different workplaces and grades, with radically contrasting terms and conditions, levels of status, opportunities and rewards. Throughout all labour markets, those occupations and professions where women predominate are valued less, paid less and deemed less skilled.

Studies which seek to document and explain the persistence of gender segregation and its characteristics have mushroomed in recent years. They include manuals on how to measure segregation (Siltanen *et al.* 1994),[2] macro studies charting patterns in the EU (Rubery and Fagan 1993), theoretical works debating the merits of competing explanations (Walby 1990), analyses of the effects of EU legislation (Duncan 1996; Hoskyns 1996; Rossilli 1997) and empirical projects in individual Member States. In the UK, for example, there are quantitative studies incorporating a range of sectors and industries (MacEwan Scott 1994) and qualitative studies looking at the social processes whereby patterns of segregation are reproduced (Cockburn 1991; Collinson *et al.* 1990). This book seeks to contribute to our understanding of this all-pervasive and persistent feature of European labour markets, but focuses on what I would argue is a neglected aspect, the role of education and training policies and practice in the reproduction of gender segregation. It looks particularly at the development of policies at the European level, and charts the evolution of approaches to delivering equal opportunities (EO) to men and women.

Systems of training provision and their take-up tend to reinforce and solidify patterns of occupational segregation. This applies to both horizontal segregation (men and women working in different industries and occupations) and vertical segregation (men and women found at different levels of the hierarchy). But vocational education and training (VET) systems are as segregated as the labour market itself. Indeed, initial, further and continuing training manifest highly gendered patterns of participation which reinforce those of the workplace. Ports of entry to further and higher education and training are modelled upon male patterns of participation in economic life, that is full-time and uninterrupted from leaving full-time education until retirement. Employer-sponsored training is concentrated upon people established in technical and managerial positions, who tend to be male. But the androcentricity of VET systems stretches far beyond mere patterns of participation. It is reflected in assumptions underpinning curricular content, funding arrangements, contact hours, location and degree of attention paid to students' and trainees' family responsibilities. It is manifested too in the informal curriculum, and the gendering of hierarchical positions among VET providers and those who set the policy agenda.

The European Commission (EC) is a major source of funding of VET within Member States through the European Social Fund (ESF), a part of the Structural Funds which comprise a package of measures set up under the Treaty of Rome in 1957 to reallocate resources to those regions most in need of economic development (see Chapter 8). Training has been supported too, during the late 1980s and early 1990s, through a series of Community Action programmes targeting particular skill development needs in the EU, for example in the new technologies (see Chapter 7). However, since the 1992 Maastricht *Treaty on European Union* became effective in 1994, the EC now has the competence to develop policies in education and training at the European level, to 'complement' the actions of individual Member States (Council of the European Community and CEC 1992). The action programmes which have been designed to deliver this European level policy are known as LEONARDO DA VINCI (for training) and SOCRATES (for education). They incorporate many of the features of the programmes which preceded them. By providing an additional source of funding for VET provision, they can potentially wield some influence on the shape and nature of activities throughout the Member States (see Chapter 8).

EEC before it, have acted as a catalyst to the reness through legislation and as a result of opean Court of Justice. Some progress has certainly been made, but there have been retrogressive steps too. While there has been some convergence on EO, the situation in different Member States remains quite varied, from Denmark and Sweden which have the most advanced policies through to Greece at the other end of the spectrum. There have been instances of EU policies leading to a levelling down in some Member States; in other words the effect of EU legislation has in some cases worsened women's position. EO has proved to be an enormously difficult objective to define, let alone deliver, and the complexity of the concept has become ever more apparent. The experiences of the Member States has thrown the inadequacies of the European to sharp relief.

e legalistic approach towards securing equal recognised and therefore complemented in the last decade by a series of positive action measures, known as the Medium Term Action Programmes on Equal Opportunities for Women and Men (see Chapter 4; CEC 1990; 1991a; 1997; Rees 1994a). These have produced examples of good practice in the field of women and work, facilitated the development of expert networks, and enabled the exchange of information. However, again, their impact falls well short of the challenge of delivering equality, largely because they focus exclusively on aspects of women's role in the labour market rather than taking a broader approach to human rights.

More recently, the idea of 'mainstreaming' equality has been the subject of debate in Brussels, prompted in part by the Fourth United Nations World Conference on the Status of Women, held in Beijing in 1995, which advocates this approach to EO in its *National Agenda for Action* (Women's National Commission *et al.* 1996). Mainstreaming involves the incorporation of EO issues into all actions, programmes and policies from the outset. It moves beyond equal treatment and positive action approaches to EO. The EC issued a potentially highly significant Communication to the Council of Ministers on incorporating EO into all Community policies and activities in 1996, a document known as the 'mainstreaming' Communication (CEC 1996). Mainstreaming involves gender monitoring and regular review of performance using gender indicators, and hence, in 1996, the Commission published its first annual report on EO: this starts to make performance in this area much more transparent than it has been in the past.

This book considers these three approaches to EO – equal treatment, positive action, and mainstreaming – within the context of the EC's policies with regard to education and training. It explores the models of EO which underpin the various policy approaches, and argues that the degree of inadequacy of the model inevitably feeds back into the effectiveness or otherwise of the approach. The book presents the argument that, while the legal framework for EO is essential, it is inevitably limited in its effectiveness. Positive action projects, while creating spaces for women and being laboratories for the development of good practice, appear to be precariously funded, provision is *ad hoc*, and there are few linkages to mainstream providers. It is mainstreaming which is likely to have the most significant impact on developing women's skills and the rigidities of gender segregation in the labour market. It also has the potential capacity to move beyond gender into other dimension of equality, such as race and disability.

EU policies on education and training and those on EO can be seen as coming together in the future due to current concerns about economic competitiveness, unemployment, social exclusion and skill shortages. Three highly significant White Papers have been produced which provide the framework for policies and action at the European level for the foreseeable future on economic, social and education and training policy at that level. While a commitment to EO is given in each of the papers, the extent to which EO informs the analysis of the problems faced, and the policies designed to address them, differs considerably. The White Papers, which are discussed in some detail in Chapter 9, are briefly introduced here in turn.

In 1994, in the context of the creation of a Single Market, an ageing workforce and chronic skill shortages, the EC published the first of the White Papers under consideration: *Growth, Competitiveness, Employment: The Challenges and Ways Forward into the 21st Century* (EC 1994a). This advocates a strategy of developing human resources to enhance competitiveness, as opposed to seeking to compete on wages. While the White Paper nods in the direction of EO, it is silent on the issue of women's training. Nevertheless, it is women who are the majority of the economically inactive and the low skilled. Women also have higher rates of unemployment and long-term unemployment in the EU. It is clearly women's skills that are most in need of developing.

In the same year, the EC produced the second White Paper, on social policy, *European Social Policy: A Way Forward for The Union* (EC 1994b). This expresses deep concern about 'social exclusion' within the EU, a concept defined largely in terms of exclusion from the labour market (see Levitas 1996). It seeks to halt processes of social and economic polarisation and identifies training as a key tool for promoting social cohesion. Women (and their children) are clearly identified in this Paper as being most at risk of poverty and social exclusion. The enhancement of women's skills is therefore seen as part of the 'way forward', and an integral component of the EU's social policy.

Training can be interpreted both as an economic policy, where the focus is on fostering the acquisition of job-related skills to develop the economy, and as a social policy, by assisting the disadvantaged to improve their occupational lifechances. It could be argued, then, that for both social and economic reasons, particularly given the focus of the policies outlined in these White Papers, the processes whereby patterns of gender segregation are perpetuated deserve intense scrutiny. Moreover, it is reasonable to expect that the social justice dimension of EO may well be emphasised rather more in the future, partly through a growing concern with human rights and partly because of the influence of Sweden (which joined the EU in 1995), given its long years of progressive policies in this field.

It is particularly timely to be considering the role of the EC in its support of VET systems and its approach to EO, given the EC's additional competencies in the field of VET conferred by the Maastricht Treaty. This has resulted in the third significant White Paper to form the backcloth to this book, this one on the subject of education and training itself: *Teaching and Learning: Towards the Learning Society* (EC 1996b). This brings together the two main arguments for upskilling the EU's workforce outlined in the economic and social White Papers (to develop economic competitiveness and to avoid social exclusion), but locates them in the context of a 'knowledge-based society'. Given the demographic structure of the Member States, with low birthrates, an ageing population and no upturn in the numbers of young recruits to the labour force anticipated until the next century (with the exception of Ireland), the shift in emphasis in training has moved from young entrants to focus upon the existing workforce, whose members will need to continue to acquire new skills throughout their working lives. The concept of 'lifelong learning' is now clearly identified in EU documentation and activities as crucial to the EU's future. The year 1996 not only saw the publication of the third White Paper but was also the European Year of Lifelong Learning, underlining the perceived increase in significance of continuing training for the development of human resources.

The book draws on research I have conducted as a consultant to the EC on EO and training policy over the last five years (see Rees 1992a; 1994a; 1994b; 1995a; 1995b; 1995c). It poses the question, to what extent do (or could) EC policies challenge the androcentricity of mainstream VET provision and related gendered patterns of segregation within the labour market of the Single Market? And is the idea of mainstreaming equality in all EU legislation and actions on VET a realistic or viable prospect? Hence, the purpose of the book is threefold. It seeks in the first instance to provide an accessible account of the role of the EU on the issue of developing EO, especially in the field of VET. Second, it offers an analysis and critique of European policy, informed by the contribution made by feminist scholars to our understanding of male dominance in culture and institutions. Finally, it engages with debates on the role of the EU in promoting economic growth, avoiding social exclusion and developing lifelong learning, the focus of the three White Papers from a gendered perspective.

The book analyses these current developments in EU policies and programmes in terms of competing concepts of EO. It seeks to trace the development of equality policies from the early days of 'equal treatment', and then 'positive action' and 'positive discrimination' through to the current discourse of 'mainstreaming equality', that is, developing a set of programmes and policies which are based on a recognition of diversity and the politics of difference. I have called these three approaches 'tinkering', 'tailoring' and 'transforming'. While equal treatment and positive action programmes have been developing over a long period, mainstreaming is a relatively new approach: competing understandings of what it entails co-exist. In the final chapter, I explore these and advocate a particular version, but, while there is growing interest in and research on mainstreaming, as yet it remains underdeveloped and largely untested.

In exploring the extent to which the EC both can and is likely to use its resources to seek to mainstream equality, the book offers both a top-down and a bottom-up analysis. In the first instance, it provides an account and critique of EO in the EC's training policies, drawing on various statistical sources, studies and documentation. In so doing it seeks to demystify the operation of the EC in this field. At the level of practice, it also draws upon the experiences of participants in EC-funded transnational projects. The clear consensus which emerges from such projects is that, while funding for individual positive action projects is welcome, the similarities in the problems faced (albeit in different regions, cultures and sectors), illustrate the need to change mainstream provision and practice. The book brings these two strands of policy and practice together in advocating a more strategic approach to training for women.

OUTLINE OF THE BOOK

The next three chapters provide a context for the more detailed empirical chapters which follow. Chapter 2 briefly outlines the industrial and socio-economic background to the book, including an account of recent patterns of gender segregation in the EU. It also provides a brief overview of the EC's education, training and equal opportunities policies. Chapter 3 focuses on deconstructing the concept of EO and outlines the conceptual framework upon which the rest of the book is based. Chapter 4 provides a history of the EC in fostering equal opportunities for men and women in the EU. This chapter (and the book itself) presumes some prior knowledge of the EU and its institutions (for good general overviews see Archer and Butler 1996; Dinan 1994; Nicholl and Salmon 1994; and Nugent 1994). The most relevant institutions and the instruments are described in the text.[3]

The next pair of chapters takes a more detailed look at the impact of training policies in one Member State, and on a particular skill shortage in the EU, that of new information technologies. Chapter 5, then, looks at gender segregation and training policy in the UK. Wales is highlighted as a European 'region' to illustrate some key issues. The skill shortages in new information technologies in the EU are discussed in Chapter 6, together with the barriers within VET systems to women filling those shortages due to the 'masculinisation of technologies'.

The final set of chapters looks at the EC and training for women in the 1990s from the macro perspective of EC training programmes. Chapter 7 draws upon primary research to provide a detailed account of the position of women in the late 1980s and early 1990s in the Community Action Programmes of the EC's Task Force Human Resources, Education, Training and Youth (TFHR, now DGXXII). These were known as ERASMUS, PETRA, LINGUA, TEMPUS, EUROTECNET, YOUTH FOR EUROPE, FORCE and COMETT. The chapter shows that the *laissez faire* approach to EO adopted in these programmes reproduced the *status quo* in terms of gender segregation. A similar story is revealed in Chapter 8, which examines the position of women in the European Social Fund and LEONARDO DA VINCI, the successor to the action programmes described in Chapter 7. The conclusion is reached that more pro-active policies are needed if the EC is not simply to reinforce, or indeed further polarise, patterns of gender segregation in level and type of skills acquired.

The final part of the book addresses the future directions of EC policies in VET and EO. Chapter 9 provides a feminist critique of the three White Papers introduced earlier in this chapter and argues that there are some contradictions between an approach which seeks to develop human capital by ensuring equal treatment of men and women on an individual approach, and policies seeking to combat social exclusion, conceived of as groups unable to compete effectively. The concluding chapter explores the conceptual, political and practical issues and agendas involved in attempts to 'feminise the mainstream'.

CONCLUSION

Despite the burgeoning literature on gender segregation in the labour market and on gender in the sociology of education, the field of training and its relationship to the reproduction of gender segregation remains relatively under-theorised. In writing this book I have attempted to bring together insights from academic literature, particularly feminist scholarship, and those from policy debates at the European level to address this issue. At the same time I seek to deconstruct some of the concepts operationalised in current thinking on the subject and demystify some of the workings of European machinery and its effects on women's training at the regional level.

Central to the book is an attempt to evaluate the effect of three different models of EO, equal treatment, positive action and mainstreaming, in education, training and labour market policy, with the emphasis on training. VET systems more appropriate to the needs of women cannot alone produce changes in the gendering of the labour market. However, a mainstreaming approach, which integrates EO into all policies, would have the potential to challenge gender segregation, by tackling the basis of the gender contract underpinned by welfare, taxation and other areas of policy as well as education, training and the labour market. The book is intended both for those interested in EO and gender studies, particularly in the context of the EU, and for those in the business of policy development and implementation.

Chapter 2

The context

The purpose of this chapter is to provide a multi-faceted context for the analysis of equal opportunities (EO) and women's training policy in the European Union (EU) which follows. The first section reviews both patterns of industrial change and continuity in the EU. The second looks at the broad picture of gender segregation in the labour force which, it is argued, training systems and structures underpin. The third section provides a brief overview of the EC's training policies, highlighting special initiatives for women. This is especially aimed at those unfamiliar with the EC's instruments for training. Much fuller accounts of these policies and analyses of their impact are provided in later chapters. The final substantive section summarises some of the main arguments for a focus on women's training in policy development which appear to have some purchase in current debates at the European level. The chapter concludes by bringing together the main strands of the context for the focus of the book.

INDUSTRIAL CHANGE

Trends in recent economic restructuring and industrial change in the EU can be seen as moving in different directions simultaneously. There are concurrent tendencies towards both globalisation and localisation. While there has been general growth in Gross Domestic Product (GDP), there has also been an increase in unemployment. Spiralling salaries among leaders of big business in certain sectors, coupled with jobless growth, has created greater gaps between those with and those without paid employment. Sustained high levels of unemployment, particularly in regions whose economic *raison d'être* has been wiped out as a result of

industrial restructuring, has led to inter-generational unemployment, while other regions appear to be in virtuous circles of
economic growth. The analysis of these, at times, countervailing
changes produces a muddled picture. This is exacerbated by what
Doogan (in press) describes as the disposition of analysts to be
preoccupied with novelty, and as a result, their tendency to under-
state continuities:

> Thus on the one hand, we are offered accounts of a virtual
> 'melt-down' of labour market institutions and practices which
> are contested by the enduring nature and longevity of many
> labour market systems. On the other hand, while poverty and
> large scale unemployment have undoubtedly assumed alarming
> proportions, we are provided with rather overblown accounts of
> the 'underclass'.

Some of these changes and continuities are explored in this section,
particularly those which have a significant gender dimension and
implications for training policy.

Whereas in the 1980s many major employers could be described
as operating a two-tier, core and peripheral, workforce where gender
played a key role in the allocation of positions, in the 1990s such
employers are more likely to have shed their peripheral functions to
small and medium-sized enterprises (SMEs) and focused on developing their core business. The highly feminised cleaning and
catering services were among the first to be contracted out (Rees
and Fielder 1992). Part-time contracts have been used increasingly,
both as a flexibility tool and as a strategy to address recruitment
difficulties (Breugal and Hegewisch 1994; Maruani 1995; Rubery *et
al.* 1995). The type of contracts available to staff in these small,
service-providing companies tends to be tenuous. Hutton (1995)
describes the ultimate in insecurity for such peripheral workers as
the 'nil-hours' contract, also known as 'on-call' work (Meulders
1995: 45), where no work is guaranteed but the worker nevertheless
is obliged to maintain their availability for the employer. Hence we
have both leaner, meaner systems of production, honed for a
competitive economy, combined with a deterioration in employees'
terms and conditions of employment and a substantial growth in
welfare bills to cater for those whose services are no longer required.

While there are many indications of an increase in the demand
for high-level skills in the knowledge-based economy (Ducatel
1994), the more pressing reality experienced in some Member States

is that there has also been a growth in low-skilled, low-paid work, for example in the caring sector (given the ageing population) and in security services (Brown 1994). The 'information society', similarly, is anticipated in terms of a mixed picture of labour demand, including new jobs, but also, fundamentally, new forms of work organisation (High Level Group of Experts 1996).

While the Single Market has not led to significant rates of human mobility across and between Member States, we are seeing substantial increases in long-term commuting and long-distance travel, such that some German cities have been described as suffering from 'thrombosis' as commuters pack the roads with private transport. Moving abroad has, however, become a fact of life for some executive grades, leading to the spawning of new businesses which specialise in relocation packages for corporate executives and their families (Deroure 1992). However, at the same time, the new technologies which allow working from home (such as teleworking) have had the effect of reducing the need for travel for some, and have created the possibility of working from the most inaccessible places while maintaining electronic communication (Huws 1995).

While some markets are global (Cooke 1996), others, particularly in the labour-intensive personal services, are highly localised. New markets are being fostered in some of the global regions, such as parts of the newly industrialised countries in eastern Europe. Meanwhile, the collapse of the Russian market has had a devastating effect on the economies of Finland and the new German Länder. Indigenous enterprises tend to respond to local markets in goods and services, but inward investment companies will sometimes also generate additional jobs in the region by utilising local supplier chains which suit just-in-time production methods. Post-Fordist methods may have been introduced into some manufacturing companies, but Fordist methods are still to be found in others (Lovering 1990), and are growing in parts of the service sector, for example in international fast food outlets, with associated low pay and poor terms and conditions of employment.

The outcome of these shifts and changes has been a significant increase in unemployment and in the number of workers whose jobs are at risk. The growth in unemployment has been identified as the single factor of greatest concern in the EU in successive policy documents (EC 1994a, 1994b). Measures are being taken to encourage employers to take on more workers through a reduction in the costs of employing staff (in the UK these costs are already much lower than elsewhere, for example Germany). Hence a deterioration in terms and conditions of employment is being advocated in order to create more jobs. However, such jobs are characteristically perilous and job gains may be transitory. Hence, while about ten million jobs were created during the period 1985–90, six million were lost in the following five years. As a consequence, in early 1995, some eighteen million people were out of work in the Single European Market, about 11 per cent of the workforce. This compares with 6.5 per cent in the United States (US) and 3 per cent in Japan (1994 figures for Japan) (EC 1995a). Moreover, the number of employees in employment declined by 4 per cent between 1991 and 1994, a drop unprecedented in the post-war period. Job losses have been particularly severe in two of the new Member States, Finland and Sweden, and in the new Länder of Germany. Table 2.1 gives some key figures on men and women and employment in the EU.

Shifts in employment by industrial sector have had implications for the balance of employment between men and women. As jobs in industry were lost during the recession of 1990–94, and services sector employment continued to grow during the same period, so the proportion of jobs in both sectors filled by women increased at a faster pace than in previous periods. Over three-quarters of women (76 per cent) and half of men (52 per cent) now work in the services sector. Some branches of this sector are overwhelmingly female, such as domestic services (90.4 per cent), health (71.8

Table 2.1. Women's and men's employment in the European Union: key figures (millions and percentages), E15, 1994[a]

	Women	Men	Total
Total population	189.9	181.1	371.1
Total employment	60.4	85.7	146.2
Activity rate (%)[b]	56.0	76.0	66.1
Self-employed (%)[c]	9.5	18.9	15.1
Employed part-time (%)[c]	30.3	4.8	15.3
Employed on a fixed-term contract (%)	12.1	10.1	11.0
Total unemployment	88.8	95.7	184.6
Unemployment rate (%)	12.8	10.0	11.1
Youth (14–24) unemployment rate (%)	21.9	20.5	21.2
Long-term unemployed (% total)[d]	48.6	45.5	47.0

Notes: [a]includes the new German Länder; [b]percentage of working-age population; [c]percentage of total employment; [d]excludes figures for Austria and Sweden
Source: Derived from EC (1995a) *Employment in Europe 1995*, Luxembourg: Office for Official Publications of the European Communities, p. 187

per cent) and education (65.4 per cent) (1992 figures) (Eurostat 1995a: 137). More and more of these jobs are part-time, even in those Member States where patterns of employment have not previously been characterised by part-time work. Hence, while women's economic activity rates have increased, this does not necessarily mean more hours are worked by women (Hakim 1993). Despite the greater job losses sustained by men, women's rate of unemployment overall in the EU (at 13 per cent) remains higher than that of men (at 10.05 per cent) (EC 1995a). While the UK has traditionally been the only Member State where the measured rate of male unemployment is higher than that of females,[1] in the enlarged Community, this situation is now also true of Finland and Sweden.

Unemployment rates throughout the EU would be higher still but for the increase in young people staying on in education and training during the period 1990–94 in all Member States except Greece and Luxembourg: this accounted for a reduction in the potential workforce size by about 3 million (EC 1995a: 11). The workforce was also diminished by a fall in the economic activity rate among older men in all Member States except Germany, Greece and Ireland. The ratio of those in employment to the population of working age in the EU (as opposed to those in the workforce, which includes the unemployed) has fallen from 62 per cent in 1992 to under 60 per cent in 1994, compared with 70 per cent in the US and 78 per cent in Japan in the same year (EC 1995a: 8). This ratio is clearly unfavourable from the perspective of sustaining a welfare system for those not in employment, such as the young, the retired and the chronically sick and disabled, as well as the unemployed. The ageing population of Europe will create additional demands upon welfare systems for the foreseeable future.

The outcome of these, at times, polar opposite trends is a highly diverse set of education, training and occupational lifechances for individuals. Workers are increasingly expected to have an adequate level of general education and the ability to learn new skills, plus the flexibility to move on to seek new training and employment in different sectors and areas when necessary. Welfare systems, not designed to cater for long-term unemployment and an ageing society, are increasingly inadequate for the task of supporting the ever-growing number of welfare dependants. Education and training systems, not designed for the growing demands of the economy for continuing training, are having to speed up the process of revision and updating of curricula and to focus on developing lifelong learning skills, rather than simply imparting a set body of knowledge or training in specific skills. Teachers, trainers and lecturers, ill-used to catering for older students and trainees, now have to adjust to students and trainees with very different profiles.

The next section examines the extent to which gender segregation is a feature of education, training and the *labour market*.

GENDER SEGREGATION

Gender segregation is increasingly recognised as a major barrier to both economic efficiency and equality in pay between men and women. Nevertheless, patterns of segregation in education, training and employment remain entrenched and, in some sectors in some Member States, are indeed worsening. A significant example here is gender segregation in the new information technologies, where the proportion of women among students enrolling in computer science degree courses, while increasing in some of the southern European States, is declining markedly in northern countries such as the UK, Germany and the Netherlands (this is discussed in more detail in Chapter 6).

Throughout the EU, there are clear differences between men and women in their patterns of take-up of post-compulsory education and training opportunities. While women are in initial training to the same extent as men, they comprise less than half the EC under-graduate population overall and considerably less than half the postgraduates. However, there has been some catching up at the undergraduate level, so that the educational qualification gap between men and women is less marked for younger age groups than for older ones. However, segregation by subject is still marked. The biggest gap between men and women by subject area is in engineering (Eurostat 1992). Women remain in a very small minority among senior staff in European universities.

Women constitute less than a third of employer-sponsored trainees on in-firm training, and are less likely to be in management posts or other senior positions where in-firm training is concentrated (Eurostat 1996). There are variations between Member States. Gender segregation in education and training in those southern European states undergoing massive restructuring and modernisation appears to be less entrenched that in some of the more stable northern European countries.

It is no surprise to find that, linked to these patterns of gender distribution in education and training systems, each Member State of the EU has a highly gendered workforce, although the specifics of the intensity and rigidity of those patterns of segregation vary. Segregation occurs at three levels: horizontally, where men and women work in different sectors; vertically, where they are found at different rungs of the ladder; and contractually, where men are more likely to have permanent full-time contracts and women to have part-time, temporary contracts (see Table 2.1), or indeed, no contracts at all (Maruani 1995).

Horizontal segregation is illustrated in Table 2.2. Women's employment has grown with the expansion of the service sector, which has been characterised by part-time work.

There are differences, but also some similarities in the extent to which certain occupations or professions are the preserve of one or other gender across Member States. Moreover, the newly industrialising eastern European countries have workforces which are just as gendered as the Member States of the EU, although some of the jobs which are regarded as being characteristically male or female are different. Recent work by Rubery and Fagan (1993) shows that patterns of gendered segregation in employment persist irrespective of changes in rates of economic activity, although, universally, more highly educated women are less likely to be economically inactive. They report:

> strong similarities in the structure of segregation by gender between countries, with low shares of women in production-related occupations and high shares in service and clerical occupations, and fairly high female shares of sales and professional occupations.
>
> (Rubery and Fagan 1993: 1)

Table 2.2.   Sectoral distribution of employment by gender, E15, 1994 (%)

	Women	Men	Total
Agriculture	4.6	6.1	5.5
Industry	17.1	40.1	30.6
Services	78.2	53.8	63.9

Source: Derived from European Commission (1995a) *Employment in Europe 1995*, Luxembourg: Office for Official Publications of the European Communities, p. 187

Of those professions expected to grow, women currently comprise only 4 per cent of senior managers, 9 per cent of engineers, and 10 per cent of high-level information technology specialists (Deroure 1993). Indeed, the rigidity of gender segregation in some of the technologically-based occupations and professions is exacerbating skills shortages in the EU in these areas (see Chapter 6).

Rubery and Fagan (1993) have charted some of the significant features of gender segregation at the EU level, and brought the figures and the trends into the public domain (see also Eurostat 1992, 1995a). They have drawn attention in particular to the position of women in 'atypical' work: part-time work, temporary contracts and 'non-employee'-status work (Rubery *et al.* 1995). This is an invaluable 'political arithmetic' exercise which is being fed into European debates on economic competitiveness. It makes ignoring the clear evidence of discriminatory practices a difficult position to sustain.

The task of explaining patterns and persistence of gender segregation in the labour force is extremely complex and is one which has engaged considerable numbers of analysts in Europe and the US for some time (see Crompton and Sanderson 1990a; van Doorne-Huiskes *et al.* 1995; MacEwan Scott 1994; Reskin and Hartmann 1986; Walby 1988). While there are many different interpretations, there is something of a consensus among many feminist theorists that the position of women in the labour market is the outcome of the interaction between the forces of patriarchy and capital, although the relative impact of these two forces, and the effect of their interaction at various stages of capitalist development, varies. The tensions and interrelations between the two systems are seen as determining the ebbs and flows of patterns of segregation, with industrial restructuring and the dynamics of labour supply and demand acting as principal catalysts.

From the supply side, it is clear that gender stereotyping in career 'choices', the ideology of the family, gendered domestic roles and power relations between men and women combine to play a significant part in determining patterns of participation. The terms upon which individual women are able to sell their labour in turn shape the type of jobs available to them. Part-time work, for example, tends overwhelmingly to be poorly paid and to offer few opportunities for training or promotion. On the demand side, employers' policies and the effect of their practices for recruitment and selection (Collinson *et al.* 1990); pay (Rubery *et al.* 1994; Sloane 1994), work organisation (Meulders 1995) and management of technology (Cockburn 1985) all contribute to the sustaining of gendered division of labour in paid work. The state also plays a role in building taxation, welfare and pension systems upon an ideology of a white nuclear family with breadwinner husband and homemaker wife, to a greater or lesser extent within the various countries of the EU. For people outside these roles, such as lesbian women and single breadwinner mothers, these sets of assumptions underpinning systems and structures make life difficult. But for all women, policies of employers and the state combine to load the dice against participation and progression along paths other than well trodden, recognisably female trajectories, which tend to be limited in range and severely truncated in promotion prospects.

Much of this is well documented. However, relatively little has been written about the impact of training systems and structures on maintaining a gendered workforce and how this interrelates with the actions of the employer and the state. In particular, given that a significant proportion of the budget of the EU is devoted to training, how do the activities funded impact upon patterns of gender segregation in the various Member States? The next section sets the scene by summarising the policy context at the EU level.

EU TRAINING POLICY AND EQUAL OPPORTUNITIES

The main resources expended by the Commission on training are allocated by the EC's Directorate-General for Employment, Industrial Relations and Social Affairs (DGV) in response to bids from authorities and organisations in the Member States through the European Social Fund (ESF), one of the arms of the EC's Structural Funds. The main aims of the ESF are to assist Member States to combat long-term and youth unemployment, and to regenerate the economies of restructuring or declining regions. The EC provides co-funding for proposals put forward by the Member States.

While an equal treatment version of EO has been enshrined in the ESF throughout its operation, at various stages in the history of the ESF funds have been earmarked for certain categories of women or to finance training and employment schemes in sectors where women were under-represented. Later reforms did not identify women as a specific target group, but it was argued that they were likely to feature strongly among the other groups identified in the priority objectives, such as the long-term unemployed and those in economically depressed regions.

However, specific attention was paid to 'women's needs' through measures launched as part of the successive Community Action Programmes on Equal Treatment of Men and Women (CEC 1991a, 1991b). A distinct shift in thinking can be detected between the first two Action Programmes, which allowed for PA projects to address the development of training for women in areas where they were under-represented, and the third Medium Term Action Programme. The latter covered the period 1991–95, and its main aim was to ' . . . entrench equality policies, and to promote women's full participation in economic and social life' (Cox 1993: 56). This is the first clear indication of a mainstreaming approach to EO, although the concept is under-operationalised in the documentation and most of the activities funded through the programme could still be described as positive action ones. For example, the Third Action Programme included the NOW (New Opportunities for Women) programme, which provides funds to Member States to promote vocational training for women, especially for the long-term unemployed and those wanting to set up in business (see CEC 1993b). NOW projects have been generally regarded as highly effective as a result of their women-centred focus, but inadequately resourced (see, for example, Callender 1994). NOW was introduced as a strand in the new Employment Community Initiative in 1995, with twice the previous budget and for a six year period. This is presented as an attempt to 'synergise' actions so that the three strands of the Employment Initiative – NOW, HORIZON (for the disabled and disadvantaged) and YOUTHSTART (for young people) – are working towards the same priorities (synergy is a much used, rarely defined Eurospeak word that suggests coordination, cross-fertilisation and complementarity). A Fourth Medium Term Action Programme has been introduced to cover the period 1996–2000, and the discourse of EO is much more clearly in the mainstreaming approach although, again, it still funds positive action projects (CEC 1995a; EC 1996a) (see Chapter 4).

IRIS, a network of women's training projects throughout the EU, is a further initiative which has been regarded as effective in identifying women's training issues and facilitating networking and opportunities for transnational learning between women's training projects (PA Cambridge Economic Consultants 1992). Jointly funded by DGV and the EC's Task Force Human Resources

Education Training and Youth (TFHR), (now DGXXII: Education, Training and Youth), the network soon established an EU-wide membership of over 500 organisations. In 1995 the IRIS network became independent of the Commission, and its members became subscribers (see Chapter 8).

In addition to the Structural Funds, in 1976 a Council of Ministers Resolution indicated it would support an action programme on education, training and youth. This was followed by Council Decisions which resulted in action programmes organised by the TFHR in the 1980s and 1990s. Rather than the 'responsive mode' mass funding of the mainstream ESF, TFHR programmes were by contrast much smaller and targeted at particular groups or designed to relieve pressure points in the development of the EU's human resources. The programmes were intended to fund innovative projects and focused on developing networks, fostering transnational partnerships and learning, and funding mobility and exchanges between teachers, students, trainers and trainees throughout the EU and, in some programmes, beyond the EU to European Free Trade Association (EFTA) countries and 'Eastern Europe'. Under Community Action programmes, support was also provided for training tools and methodologies, especially in new technologies, fostering university enterprise links, and training trainers (see Chapter 7, and CEC 1989, 1991c, 1992, 1993b, 1993c for full descriptions of programmes and their projects and activities).

Following the Maastricht Treaty, LEONARDO DA VINCI and SOCRATES were introduced to build upon and supersede these programmes. The intention was to provide more streamlined, focused programmes to allow more 'synergy', LEONARDO bringing together training activities and SOCRATES those of education. The old programmes can be traced through to new identities as strands or sub-strands in the new programmes.

LEONARDO DA VINCI has three strands: improving the quality of vocational training provision; encouraging innovation in training methods; and developing the European dimension at all levels. SOCRATES extends the EU's action to all levels of education including secondary schools, higher education and teacher training. Its three strands promote cooperation between higher education (as before, under ERASMUS); encourage partnership between secondary schools; and develop horizontal activities targeting all levels of education. This will include open and distance learning, language learning and exchanges of experience.

The original programmes all referred to the principle of equal treatment of men and women in the Council Decisions which set them up, but as Chapter 7 shows, this *laissez faire* approach to EO resulted in a pattern of participation in the programmes which reinforced existing gender divisions. For example, while there were almost equal numbers of men and women in PETRA, the initial training programme aimed at young people, women were relatively sparse in the more technologically based training programmes such as FORCE and COMETT. In LEONARDO and SOCRATES, a more pro-active encouragement of EO is slowly being built into the application and selection procedures, and the monitoring and evaluation systems (see Chapter 8).

WOMEN AND EC TRAINING POLICIES

The current combination of economic and social factors has focused attention on occupational gender segregation, which is now regarded by both the Commission and the 'Social Dialogue' of employers' and unions' representatives in Brussels as an important policy issue. Moreover, the Essen Summit of the Council of Ministers in 1995 identified as the two main objectives for future action combating unemployment and equal opportunities for men and women. These two are linked: the drive for gender equality is seen through an economic 'prism' (Duncan 1996: 411) which focuses on the fight against unemployment and the drive for economic competitiveness.

The Single European Market and the enhanced powers afforded the EU in the field of vocational education and training (VET) in the Maastricht Treaty have meant the Commission increasingly has scope to develop education and training policy at the EU level. Article 126 underlines the role of the Union in contributing to the development of high quality education, while Article 127 allows a vocational training policy to be developed at EU level for the first time to support and supplement the action of the Member States. LEONARDO DA VINCI and SOCRATES are the action programmes designed to assist the Commission fulfil these additional responsibilities. The three White papers, on economic (EC 1994a), social (EC 1994b) and teaching and learning policy (EC 1996b) spell out the approaches to be taken in meeting the skills needs of the EU. To what extent do such policy documents focus on the development of women's skills?

The message of the economic White Paper is that, given growing international competition with some low-skill, low-labour-cost Pacific rim countries in particular,[2] there is a perceived need for the EU's labour force to focus on high quality market niche goods and services. This implies making the most of human resources by developing high-level skills and qualifications. The workforce needs to be adaptable, to develop good communication and diagnostic skills, and to be capable of teamworking and lifelong learning (CEC 1993d).

Training systems, therefore, are seen as needing to gear up for these new imperatives to avoid skills shortages. The concept of skill is of course socially constructed (Gaskell 1986) and highly gendered. Von Prondzynski (1986) points to the way in which 'feminine skills' (such as manual dexterity and speed) are valued less than alleged 'masculine' qualities (such as physical strength) in collective agreements and judicial decisions. The concept of skill shortages is equally problematic (see Green and Ashton 1989 for a distinction between skill deficits and skill shortages). Nevertheless, the widespread belief that skills shortages are already threatening the economic competitiveness of the EU has been an important motivator in the development of training policies. The Industrial and Development Advisory Committee of the Commission of the European Communities, made up largely of leading industrialists, produced an influential report on skill shortages in Europe (IRDAC 1991) and the Social Partners have expressed concern about skill needs in their *Joint Opinion on Women and Training* (CEC and Social Dialogue 1993).[3] The Commission too has drawn attention to the issue, particularly skill shortages in the knowledge-based industries, which are seen as being the cornerstone of the EU's market (Ducatel 1994; CEC 1993d).

General trends observable in the process of industrial restructuring have led such observers to predict a net increase in the demand for skills, even in those occupations not historically associated with training and skill development. The all-pervasiveness of new information technologies gives them a momentum of their own in the demand for training and skills. Even those in occupations and professions not traditionally associated with new technologies, such as nurses and hotel receptionists, are increasingly required to operate spreadsheets or to be skilled in telecommunications. Similarly, the growing emphasis on the delivery of good-quality goods and services, and ensuring high levels of customer satisfaction, arguably entails enhanced training for all workers.

The development of women's skills is seen as essential to meet the changing skill needs. They comprise, after all, the majority of the economically inactive, sometimes described as the 'latent workforce'; those neither in work nor looking for work, but who emerge when new jobs with flexible hours are offered in the locality, for example when a new supermarket is opened. Given the projected increase in the demand for labour at a time when the number of school-leavers is set to decline, more employers will be seeking to recruit such women. The largest category is likely to be women returning to work after a period at home, with outdated skills and, potentially, eroded self-confidence. Given the correlation between economic activity and high levels of education (Rubery and Fagan 1993), such women are likely to have intermediate, low-level, out of date or no qualifications.

There are of course cultural differences in the extent to which some categories of women engage in paid work. Married women and mothers in France are more likely to be in paid employment than those in Germany (Fagnani 1996). Indeed, in Germany, the breadwinner/homemaker ideology underpins a highly conservative welfare system which makes it difficult for married women with children to participate in the labour force on a full-time basis. Even the childcare facilities are designed to assist such women with their domestic responsibilities rather than participate in paid work (Duncan 1996). This contrasts with Denmark where the taxation and benefit structure combine with childcare provision to enable women to participate in the workforce on a much more equal basis. In southern regions of Mediterranean Member States such as Portugal, Spain, Italy and Greece, many women do not engage in paid work because it is socially unacceptable for them to be seen in public in that capacity (see Delamont 1994, chapter 9). Nevertheless, changes in these economies, and in particular the growth of hospitality industries, mean that even here, new labour market entrants are increasingly likely to include women (Castelberg-Koulma 1991; Rees 1994d). Moreover, the restructuring of the education system in Spain and Portugal has enabled well educated, middle class women to gain higher-level qualifications. Changing attitudes in these countries have facilitated well qualified, professional women to progress (Duncan 1996).

Women employees tend to be segregated in low-skilled work in organisations which currently offer no opportunities for upskilling: secretarial and clerical workers are the most obvious examples here. Existing part-time workers may wish to extend their hours and skills. Women in middle management could be trained to fill the growing demand for senior management staff. Female-dominated sectors, such as tourism, retail, caring and catering tend to be perceived as low-skilled and are seen as a potential focus of training initiatives at all levels, given the increased pressure on achieving high-quality standards to ensure international competitiveness.

Finally, women wanting to become self-employed, to contribute to family businesses, or to set up their own businesses, have also been identified as targets for training, especially in regions which are depressed or undergoing industrial restructuring (CEC 1987a; May 1987). The majority of new small enterprises set up in the 1980s were started by women (CEC 1993b). There has been special attention paid to 'helper spouses', that invisible army of workers, for the most part women, who assist their partners in their small business, be it a small-holding or general medical practice, who have tended hitherto not to have had employment protection or access to training (Finch 1983; Hunt 1993). Local employment initiatives are an important arm of regional economic development.

It can be argued, then, that women comprise the majority of those in need of training among each of the constituent parts of the labour force: in addition to being the vast majority of new labour force entrants (OECD 1994), they have higher rates than men both of unemployment and of long-term unemployment (Eurostat 1995a, see Table 2.1), and they are the majority of the low-skilled among employees and the self-employed. All these groups tend to be without educational qualifications in an era of growing credentialism.

In addition to these economic reasons for the focus on women's training, the feminisation of poverty and long-term unemployment in the EU have sharpened the social and hence the political focus: the position taken in the EC's Social Policy White Paper is that women's training needs must be met if they and their children are to avoid poverty and social exclusion (EC 1994b). This has added fuel to the political imperative to address women's training as a policy issue.

CONCLUSION

There have undoubtedly been some profound changes in the labour market of the EU in recent years, and yet there have been significant continuities at the same time, one of the most robust of which is that the labour market is segregated by gender. Despite patterns of industrial restructuring, the shift towards service sector employment, the growth in atypical work and the increasing influence of new technologies in shaping jobs, gender remains the most significant determinant of occupational lifechances. As the effects of developments in capitalism are felt in labour market changes, so patriarchy, like modelling clay, reshapes itself. The cards for the new economic order are dealt, and women are yet again to be found in the jobs with least training, poorer pay and least favourable contracts.

The EC and Social Partners look closely to competing economies for comparison of performance and have identified the development of a skill-based workforce as the way forward. In some senses, women are seen as the weak link. With qualifications less relevant to labour market needs, and forming the majority of the low-skilled members of the existing and future workforce, a new political imperative has focused attention on women's training needs, and the EU's need for trained women. While this not a universally held analysis, it is sufficiently influential to feed through to key policy documents and the design of a series of measures aimed at developing a skilled workforce. This has acted as a catalyst in taking EO more seriously. It is no longer seen as just a social justice issue, but increasingly as an economic imperative. The next chapter traces the approach from equal treatment in the Treaty of Rome, through positive action in the 1980s, to the mainstreaming agenda of the 1990s.

Chapter 3

Conceptualising equal opportunities

A cartoon shows a man behind a desk in a jungle clearing addressing a line-up of various creatures – cat, monkey, elephant, sea-lion, snake, frog, bird and a goldfish in a bowl on a pedestal. 'To ensure a fair selection you all get the same test' he says. 'You must all climb that tree.'
(DGXXII (1995) *Alpha Toolkit: Make changes for today which will be solutions for tomorrow*, Brussels: DGXXII European Commission p. 25)

The concept of equal opportunities is riddled with problematic constructs. Policies aimed at achieving EO are, by the same token, deeply fraught and tend to be limited in their effectiveness. Rooted in ideologies about the nature of a 'just society', competing and at times contradictory underlying assumptions are rarely thoroughly questioned or examined by organisations committed to being 'equal opportunities employers'. Added to this complexity is the tension in the relationship between EO principles and the workings of a *laissez faire* labour market. Some commentators argue that policies designed to achieve EO are an expensive luxury and at odds with the operation of an efficient economy. Others maintain that to have the distribution of positions within hierarchies (and indeed the structuring of organisations themselves) influenced by ascriptive (inherited) characteristics such as gender and race rather than by merit is economically inefficient and supremely wasteful of human resources. Moreover, it is argued, in the context of the global economy, it is precisely the efficient use of human resources which provides a competitive edge.

This chapter scrutinises some of these issues and outlines a range of approaches towards EO. Beginning with liberal philosophical thinking about equal treatment and equality of access, it moves on to examine concerns about equality of outcome, and positive action and positive discrimination. Finally it looks at more recent ideas about deconstructing the underlying orientations of organisations, such as their androcentricity (or 'male-centredness') and Eurocentrism, and the way they operate to the advantage of stake-holders, reproducing elites who share common characteristics in dimensions of gender, class and race. This leads to a consideration of those policies which seek to 'mainstream' EO which are based on the 'politics of difference'. They seek to transform organisations and create a culture of diversity in which people of a much broader range of characteristics and backgrounds may contribute and flourish. This potentially has the advantage not simply of widening the gender base of organisations but also of tackling other forms of disadvantage and discrimination, on the grounds of race, ethnic origin, nationality, disability, sexual orientation and regional, linguistic and cultural difference. There are, however, competing understandings of the mainstreaming approach, some of which would almost certainly have deleterious effects for EO.

Much has been written on how language affects the social construction of male and female subjectivity (Violi 1992; Weedon 1987) and how co-existing discourses have different statuses in rela-tion to each other (Foucault 1980). In discussions of EO, a set of key concepts recurs, most of which have a variety of meanings and usages. This is at the root of some of the difficulties in devising effective policies in education, training and employment. These terms include equality, equity, fairness, sameness, difference, just, justice, disadvantage, and discrimination. There are many helpful, detailed discussions, both of meanings of these terms and of their implications for effective delivery of EO policies (see for example Brah 1991; Brine 1995a; Cockburn 1989, 1991; Jewson and Mason 1986; Maynard 1994; Phillips 1987; Webb and Liff 1988; Young 1990). The purpose of this chapter is to draw attention to the main conceptual approaches and to offer working definitions for inter-pretations of accounts which follow.

The discourse of EO gives rise to many interpretations, not simply by different actors sharing the same language but in transna-tional debates. Such debates at the European level illustrate the variation in the extent to which the languages of the Member States share (or rather, fail to share) a common set of concepts and the words to describe them. In some languages, for example Flemish and Swedish, there is no satisfactory translation for the word 'gender'. This can give rise to confusion in transnational discussions where a distinction needs to be made between biological (sex) and socially constructed (gender) differences between men and women. In Spanish, 'positive action' is translated as 'positive discrimination', despite the distinct conceptual difference in meaning in English and other languages (see below). Employers seeking to keep within the law on equal treatment when drafting job advertisements face particular challenges if the language they use is a gendered one. Indeed, the Equal Opportunities Commission (EOC) has found it necessary to publish guidelines for employers advertising in Welsh, given that the language has no female versions of some job titles (Awbery 1997). The gendering of concepts more generally creates difficulties for the analysis of EO in education, training and the labour market. This issue is taken up in Chapter 5 with regard to the English language, where concepts such as skill and unemployment are shown to be gendered in their social construction. This has a series of implications for the analysis, understanding and development of policy. Mapping terms and concepts concerned with EO at the European level is clearly a vital task in the mainstreaming agenda.[1]

After discussion of three broad approaches to EO (equal treatment, positive action and discrimination, and politics of difference), the chapter offers corresponding models of EO approaches in training policy, characterised as 'tinkering', 'tailoring' and 'transforming'. Tinkering can be roughly equated to liberal approaches to equal treatment (resting on the notion of 'sameness'), while tailoring seeks to integrate women into organisations and cultures structured around the needs of men, by making special provision for the ways in which they are 'different' from men. However, transforming acknowledges the differences among men as well as those among women, and, by recasting mainstream provision, seeks to accommodate both gender and other dimensions of discrimination and disadvantage, for example those based on ethnicity and disability.

This conceptualisation of models of EO forms the theoretical framework of critiques of EO policies in relation to training strategies at the European level for the rest of the book. The empirical chapters which follow seek to illustrate the limitation of equal treatment and positive action approaches in training policy and argue the need for a transformative approach.

EQUAL TREATMENT

The concept of equality of opportunity constructed as equal treatment or equal access for women arguably traces its roots to Mary Wollstonecraft (1967 [1792]) and the liberal feminist tradition. She extended the notion of citizens' rights, debated by philosophers such as Jean Jacques Rousseau at the time of the French Revolution, to include those of women (although she focused exclusively on middle class women: like many Enlightenment writers of the time, her notion of equal rights did not extend across class boundaries). Fundamentally the concept of equality implies that no individual should have fewer human rights or opportunities than any other. It is a concept that few but the most extreme now have difficulty in supporting, at least in principle.

However, if the intention is to challenge the significance of certain ascribed characteristics in determining the allocation of positions, then the main problem with the equal treatment approach to EO is simply that it is ineffective. This is unsurprising. It will inevitably reproduce inequalities that exist in the broader context. The systems and structures which perpetuate unequal power relations between men and women (and between people from different classes or races) as groups in wider society inevitably impact upon organisations seeking to offer 'equal treatment' to men and women.

The weakness of the equal treatment approach lies in a lack of analysis of the relationship between public and private spheres. In effect, public life is ring-fenced as if it were unaffected by inequalities in the arena of private life. As Humm (1989: 63) has argued:

> even with the granting of equality to women in public life, women's domestic labour will always be unequal to that of men. More subtly, the hidden patriarchal agendas of public institutions can subvert the apparent equality of legal rights.

There are clear connections articulated here between patterns of inequality in the private sphere and those which then result in the public sphere. Granting equal access to men and women will only benefit certain women: those whose cultural capital, experiences, family circumstances and share of domestic responsibilities are similar to those of men as a group.

The equal treatment model is rooted, then, in a narrow distributive conception of justice, and focuses the debate upon the allocation of positions within a hierarchy which is given. It ignores the impact of patriarchy in the home and its interaction with capital to produce gendered organisations which systematically disadvantage women. It discounts the impact of other forms of unequal power relations, for example those which accrue as a result of class or racial oppression and discrimination. Systematic domination of some groups by others is reflected in organisational institutions, systems and structures. The equal treatment approach simply removes the more obvious structural barriers to individuals' access to systems which themselves are shaped by those patterns of domination and oppression.

The ineffectiveness of equal treatment as a model of EO policy is illustrated by the highly gendered patterns of segregation operating within the professions in the UK to which women have technically been granted 'equal access'. In the nineteenth and early twentieth centuries, women were legally prohibited from becoming qualified in the major professions such as law and accountancy. Legislation banning the exclusion of women from the professions was finally passed in the 1919 *Sex Disqualification (Removal) Act*. While women began to enter these professions, it remained legal to pay them different rates and to discriminate against them on the grounds of gender. Women civil servants were obliged to resign on marriage in Northern Ireland up until 1972. The *Sex Discrimination Act* and *Equal Pay Act* passed in the 1970s and brought into effect in 1975 made it illegal to discriminate on the grounds of sex in education, training, employment and pay. The EOC was set up at that time to monitor the law and suggest amendments, to foster the development of EO for men and women, and to back legal cases of discrimination brought by individuals and groups.[2]

In the 1980s and 1990s, women have been entering training for the professions in increasingly substantial numbers, aided by this legislation and by the transparency and qualifications-based specificity of entry requirements. As Crompton (1987) argues, it is more difficult to discriminate directly against the entry of members of a specific group into training for professions which operate a qualifications lever for entry. By contrast, it is noticeable that women have not made the same inroads into senior management positions in the UK, particularly in the private sector (Hansard Society Commission on Women at the Top 1990; McRae 1996) where routes of entry are not as transparent and are less linked to the acquisition of specific qualifications, and where networks are far more significant in the allocation of posts (Coe 1992).

Women now constitute about half the undergraduates on courses for the professions in the UK. However, gaining equal access to courses has not resulted in the disappearance of gender as an organising principle in the allocation of positions within professions (see Atkinson and Delamont 1990 for a general account of female marginality in the learned occupations; see also Allen (1988) on medicine; Fogarty *et al.* (1981) on the civil service, architecture and industry; Spencer and Podmore (1987) on law, medicine, health service administration and engineering; and West and Lyon (1995) on academia). Women are clustered in certain fields within the professions. In medicine, for example, they are found in general practice and community medicine, while in law, they are likely to focus on family and divorce law or work in the public rather than the private sector which tends to offer more flexible work conditions and return to work arrangements, if not better salaries. In academic life, women are concentrated in contract research posts. Even the 3.5 per cent (1989/90) of professors in the UK who are women earn considerably less than their male counterparts after holding constant age and years of service (Association of University Teachers 1992; West and Lyon 1995).

This shift from exclusion from certain spheres of public life to segregation within it (Walby 1990) represents the fall-out of the interaction between patriarchy and capitalism. The interests of both systems co-determine certain prescribed and limited terms on which women may enter and progress within the professions. Few are found in senior positions in the professional associations which shape the agenda and determine the nature of the hurdles for admission and progression. Overwhelming evidence suggests that there have not been major shifts in the domestic division of labour despite the increase in female economic activity rates (Brannen and Moss 1991; Morris 1990; Pahl 1984; Warde and Hetherington 1993; Witherspoon 1988). The group which is particularly heavily burdened comprises those women with part-time jobs, who tend to have young children and are either single parents (Dex 1988) or receive very little assistance from their partners (Gershuny *et al.* 1986, 1994). Hence only some women in some circumstances can compete on equal terms with men. Their ability to do so is cited as evidence that equal access exists for those who wish to take advantage of it. In reality, such equality of access is an illusion. In addition to unequal demands made on the time of men and women for domestic responsibilities, a variety of exclusionary mechanisms, experienced by women as 'chill factors', still operate widely within the professions inhibiting women from reaching the top jobs (see, for example, Rees *et al.* [in press] on women and principal posts in Northern Ireland).

Walby (1990) and Duncan (1996) draw attention to the significance of societal 'gender contracts' between men and women which are underpinned by taxation, welfare, childcare and other institutional arrangements. Gender contracts are defined by Duncan as 'a rough social consensus on what women and men do, think and are' (1996: 415). They inform expectations about the domestic division of labour and power relations which, in turn, shape systems and structures that reinforce those expectations. These combine to exercise a strong influence on economic activity rates and patterns of gender segregation. While Duncan argues that the nature of the gender contract for any society can change, such patterns tend to be relatively long lasting. Equality policies, such as the provision of childcare, that do not address underlying gender contracts will inevitably be limited in their effects.

This is demonstrated in the review of EO measures which follows. A legal framework providing for equal treatment for men and women is clearly essential; however, this approach focuses on the establishment of rights and procedures rather than on outcomes. One of the main criticisms of the shortcomings of European law on EO is that it focuses on issues of equal treatment of men and women as workers, hence it leaves the inequalities rooted in the gender contract largely untouched. In other words, it addresses the symptoms rather than the causes of inequality. As a consequence, it is clearly limited in its potential effectiveness.

In the UK, equal treatment legislation has clearly had some effect on the position of women in education, training and employment. However, it was the 1944 Education Act, principally designed to provide free and compulsory education for all children aged between five and fourteen as a device to open up higher education opportunities to children from the working class, which enabled girls to have equal access to education for the first time. However, this equal access to education nevertheless still had the effect of reinforcing the gender contract, as the curriculum was designed to gear children to their future roles in the sexual division of labour: girls as homemakers and boys as breadwinners (EOC 1996a).[3]

EC Directives led to the introduction of EO legislation to make sex discrimination in employment and pay unlawful all in the

Member States in the 1970s; similar legislation had been introduced in the UK by the Labour Government in 1970. However, despite the one-off reduction in the pay differential between men and women following the Equal Pay Act, the impact of legislation has been highly circumscribed (Gregory 1987, 1992; Kahn and Meehan 1992; Leonard 1987a, 1987b; Rubery *et al.* 1994). Patterns of vertical and horizontal segregation remain cemented both within education and training systems and in the labour force. The impact of the original Equal Pay Act (not brought into effect until 1975 to allow employers time to get their house in order) was undermined by patterns of gender segregation which meant women had no male 'comparator' with whom to claim equal pay. The Equal Pay for Work of Equal Value (1984) amendment, introduced to address this issue, has had limited effect because of the cultural barriers attached to valuing work largely done by women in the same terms as that done by men (Kahn and Meehan 1992). Von Prondzynski (1986) points to the way in which 'feminine skills' (such as manual dexterity and speed) are valued less than alleged 'masculine' qualities (such as physical strength) in collective agreements and judicial decisions. The personal and financial cost of bringing action inhibits the widespread use of the law to further EO (Leonard 1987b) and the limited resources available to the EOC means that support has to be restricted to cases deemed winnable which further clarify or extend the law.

Equality of access (*égalité des chances*) clearly does not lead in practice to equality of outcome (*égalité des faits*). The concept of EO as a necessary and sufficient measure to eliminate the impact of gender on educational and employment lifechances is therefore found wanting. Equal treatment legislation has not significantly affected either the rigidities of segregation within occupations and professions, nor has it eliminated (although it has clearly diminished) gendered differentials in pay. Indeed, as we shall see in Chapter 7 on the impact of EC action programmes on training for women, equal treatment policies can in some circumstances reinforce the *status quo*, or, indeed, even increase skill gaps between men and women.

A further weakness in the equal treatment approach lies in the passive approach to the application of the principle. Equal treatment policies are not always reinforced by any mechanisms to ensure their application or to monitor performance. A statement to the effect that an organisation has an EO policy is clearly not sufficient to ensure its application. Pro-active procedures, such as gender monitoring, awareness-raising and training at the very least, are necessary to make equal treatment effective within its own limited terms. The work of Cockburn (1991) and Collinson *et al.* (1990) has been extremely important in using qualitative field work to dissect the processes by which organisations reproduce their cultures (including the characteristics of individuals in positions within hierarchies), even when equal treatment policies of varying strengths are in place.

The failure of equal treatment to produce equal outcome lies, then, in the lack of analysis of the causes of segregation, be it along gender, race or any other dimension. The failure to acknowledge the impact of hierarchies such as patriarchal ordering through the gender contract, and racial oppression, limits the scope of equal treatment actions. The equal treatment approach suggests that people should be treated simply as individuals without recognising the impact of group membership in the allocation of positions and the implications of this for cultural reproduction. It is limited, too, by weak application of the principle. Positive action and positive discrimination measures have been introduced in many settings to seek to address this weakness.

POSITIVE ACTION AND POSITIVE DISCRIMINATION

Positive action

The concept of positive action (PA) recognises that equal treatment can reinforce existing inequalities. PA measures seek (in the hackneyed phrases) 'to create a level playing field' or 'to untie the hand behind women's backs'. The emphasis shifts from equality of access to creating conditions more likely to result in equality of outcome by equalising starting positions. The notion of merit determining outcome is still in place and the terms by which merit is defined remain unquestioned. The contribution of PA is to assist women to compete more effectively within the existing construction of merit.

PA rests on the notion that membership of groups makes a difference to outcome. PA measures have been based on attempts to identify barriers to women's participation in education, training and employment. They seek to provide mechanisms which will facilitate women's entry on an equal footing by compensating for unequal starting positions. They are predicated on addressing the ways in which women are 'different' from men and thereby 'disadvantaged'. This approach begins, then, with a recognition of the significance of group membership determined by ascriptive characteristics in the allocation of positions. It acknowledges the dominance and oppression of some groups by others. Like equal treatment, however, it is principally concerned with the distribution of positions within hierarchies rather than with challenging the structural *status quo* which reinforces systems of oppression in those hierarchies.

Women-only management training courses provide an example of PA training for women which in some cases is designed to assist them to behave more like a man or to survive in a male culture. Curricula headings include 'developing a killer instinct', 'coping with the office romeo', 'making yourself heard in meetings'. Such training, while much appreciated by course participants, and deemed effective by them in assisting promotion prospects, seeks to adapt women to a particular model of masculinity dominant in management hierarchies (Pollert and Rees 1992; Tanton 1994). There can be casualties from this approach. Marshall (1995) for example documents the case of women senior managers who drop out not because of the work but because of their discomfiture within a male dominated culture.

One of the best known PA measures in employment is the UK's Opportunity 2000, launched by Business in the Community and backed by the (then) Prime Minister, the Rt Hon Mr John Major. Signatories to Opportunity 2000 are, for the most part, a group of large employers who are publicly committed to improving *inter alia* the proportion of women in middle management and top jobs through various forms of PA. Many of these employers conducted an analysis of the gender make-up of their workforce, introduced actions such as EO awareness raising, appointed an EO officer, and set goals and targets for proportions of women in certain grades by the year 2000. Progress is being monitored, but annual reports of Business in the Community suggest, unsurprisingly, that change is slow. The recession is identified as causing difficulties in sustaining momentum (Business in the Community 1992, 1993; Hammond 1992).

However, more deep-seated, structural and attitudinal factors may also be at work. Hammond and Holten (1991) suggest that, to be effective, PA measures need commitment from the top, widespread 'ownership' of the policy (whereby all employees and especially line managers are committed to it and share responsibility for it), links with business plans, and adequate resources. This package of support measures is rarely systematically applied. Voluntary PA measures do not on the whole deliver the cultural and organisational change required to combat gender segregation. A number of qualitative studies have documented all too graphically the mechanisms used by line managers to subvert such policies and the way in which male backlash can erupt in organisations seeking to develop PA (Cockburn 1989, 1991).

In training, PA measures which seek to address gender inequalities aim to establish the extent to which gender is an issue, and then to adapt provision to take on board women's 'special position'. This may arise because of their career breaks, their domestic commitments, or because they are under-represented in certain subjects and at some levels. Hence PA in training includes measures to accommodate women's domestic responsibilities, to check for gender biases in course materials, and to provide special supplementary training (for example for women wanting to enter construction industry trades) to make up the 'deficit' of their knowledge compared with that of men before they begin a mainstream training course. Women-only training by women tutors, especially for women returning to work or entering training in male-dominated fields, is also categorised as a PA training measure. Such courses characteristically include assertiveness training for women (see Willis and Daisley 1990). These measures are discussed in more detail later in this chapter.

Awareness raising is an important aspect of PA measures. The Government- and EOC-backed UK Fair Play initiative, which was started as a grass roots movement in Wales as *Chwarae Teg* (Welsh for 'fair play'), comprises regionally-based consortia of organisations which seek to raise awareness of the barriers to women's participation in work both qualitatively and quantitatively (DfEE/EOC 1997). The initiative has already spread to Belgium and the Netherlands, and there are plans to set up Fair Play in Italy and a number of other Member States. Much of the emphasis in Fair Play is on raising awareness of the need to develop women's skills, to address the issue of childcare needs, and to recognise and remove barriers to women's recruitment and progression in the workplace.

In Belgium, the Netherlands and Italy, some PA programmes are backed by the force of law, and financial incentives accrue to employers providing such programmes from the State. In Italy, France and Belgium, there are collective agreements between employers' and trade unions' organisations on women's training. In parts of the US, PA is enforced by contract compliance. There is very little PA training in the UK, where such actions are voluntary, and, indeed, of all EU Member States, the UK is the only one which still places restrictions on certain categories of women taking up training opportunities for the unemployed because of their ineligibility for unemployment benefit in their own right.[4] While it is possible to apply for exemption under the *Sex Discrimination Act* to provide single-sex training, this facility is under-used as a mechanism to train women in areas where they are under-represented.

Positive discrimination

It can be argued that equal treatment is in itself in effect discriminatory, given the different sets of cultural capital and normative expectations of men and women and the history of discrimination and disadvantage. PA can be seen as providing window dressing; it facilitates some women in some areas, in particular well qualified, middle class women seeking to enter the professions, without affecting the *status quo* for the vast majority. It does not challenge the culture and structure of organisations which give rise to inequalities in the first place. Different treatment according to different circumstances is needed, the argument runs, to ensure not simply equality of opportunity but equality of outcome. The policy implication of this analysis is positive discrimination (PD).

PD seeks to bring about changes to the *status quo* through mechanisms designed to increase the participation of the under-represented group: it is in effect the application of 'unequal treatment'. In the US, affirmative action measures allow for positive discrimination in some areas of employment in favour of women and members of ethnic minorities. Quotas also operate in Sweden. This approach is seen as a temporary measure to even up the balance of characteristics, such as gender and race, of people in sectors or at levels in the hierarchy which are particularly skewed. PD in employment is illegal in the UK.

PD thus goes further than PA. It acknowledges that discrimination exists and needs to be addressed: it seeks to redress uneven balances. Discrimination can be active or passive. Failure to know about the relationship between characteristics in the distribution of resources or positions is interpreted as passive discrimination. Failure to undertake gender (or ethnic) monitoring has been identified therefore as a form of passive discrimination. Organisations that are contractually bound to show that they are offering equal treatment to groups in their provision need to monitor their performance of services to be aware of the outcomes of their actions.

This was shown graphically in an evaluation of the extent to which the Training and Enterprise Councils in England and Wales, charged in their contracts with providing equal treatment for ethnic minorities, were found guilty of passive discrimination by not having instigated ethnic monitoring (Boddy 1995). Boddy argues that key elements in combating discrimination, once monitoring has illustrated the pattern of outputs, are a diagnosis of causes, and evaluation and feedback linked into subsequent action. This rarely happens. TECs have also been the subject of a formal investigation by the EOC which revealed many had inadequate mechanisms for gender monitoring (EOC 1993).

The key question is, what should EO policies set out to achieve? Should they move beyond equal treatment to counterbalance the effects of past discrimination? In 1996, the British Labour Party decided that, in order to increase the low and apparently declining number of women in the House of Commons, it was necessary to produce all-women short lists for nominated candidates in certain seats where new candidates were being selected, with the agreement of the local party. This produced both considerable backlash and some vehement support. Comments from those opposed to this form of PD couched their objections in terms of the desirability to have 'equal treatment' of candidates and not to 'discriminate' on the grounds of gender. Such arguments were highly revealing in showing the models of equality within which the protagonists were operating. The exercise provoked considerable hostility and its legality was successfully contested.

A problematic issue in PD is that of the gendering of value. It is difficult to engender parity of esteem for activities and occupations that are valued differently because of their gendered associations. Campaigns for equal pay for work of equal value have argued that, while women's jobs may be different from those of men, nevertheless they can be equally demanding, and have an equivalence in level of skill required (Kahn 1992). This moves the debate on from the concept of sameness to recognising and establishing equivalence, and, by implication, the need to seek parity of esteem and reward for different, gendered activities (Kahn and Meehan 1992). Job evaluation schemes provide an underused opportunity to deconstruct the skill levels of various occupations irrespective of the usual gender of the occupants.

A further dimension of equality is the concept of indirect discrimination, the most obvious example of which was the situation in the UK where part-time workers were not entitled to employment benefits (such as employment protection, redundancy entitlements and maternity rights) on the same basis as full-time workers. As the vast majority of part-time workers are women, this was eventually recognised as indirect discrimination and, despite considerable vociferous objections from the business world, was eventually addressed through equal treatment legislation enforced on the UK by a European Directive.

Policies towards EO, then, can be permissive, they can include PA measures based on an analysis of the 'barriers' facing women, or they can be discriminatory – that is, they can positively favour a less represented group in order to achieve a better balance. However, these approaches to EO, which seek to ensure equality of access and which address disadvantages in certain groups, can only go so far in bringing about equality of outcome. Such 'procedural' models (West and Lyon 1995) focus on the elimination of discriminatory practices so that 'merit' will apparently determine who rises to the top. But as Young (1990) has argued, such systems leave unquestioned an hierarchical division of labour and a supposed allocation of people to top places on the grounds of merit. Young asserts that the notion of merit as measured by the applications of impartial measures of technical competence is a myth. Moreover, affirmative (positive) action challenges principles of liberal equality and represents the application of the distributive paradigm of justice:

> It defines racial and gender justice in terms of the distribution of privileged positions among groups, and fails to bring into question issues of institutional organization and decision making power.
>
> (Young 1990: 193)

This brings us to what West and Lyon (1995) describe as the structural model which takes issue with organisational arrangements that are regarded as constructing barriers and impediments to the benefit of one group more than another. The procedural model which underpins positive action focuses on the elimination of informal discriminatory practices so that imbalances in opportunities are redressed and 'merit' will then determine who rises to the top. Positive discrimination seeks to 'correct' the distribution of positions by a system of quotas to create a 'fairer balance'. However, the more radical structural model is concerned with effecting outcomes by changing cultures, and thereby systems and structures, rather than perfecting or skewing the rules of the contest. It has the potential to address the gender contract underpinning systems and structures. The next section examines the structural model which I have called mainstreaming.

MAINSTREAMING EQUALITY

The model of EO which underlies mainstreaming policies is based upon the notion of the politics of difference. While the significance of the concept of difference between groups rather than sameness among individuals is now widely accepted, its implications for policies seeking to ensure EO are less well understood. Squires (1994: 7) shows how this is due to a confusion between the importance of difference and domination:

> we need to ask of equal opportunities whether it is difference or disadvantage which is our primary concern, for there is a difference between distinguishing people according to group attributes, and explicitly restricting the actions and opportunities of group members. Yet simple difference all too often does translate into perceived inferiority. . . . Of central importance . . . is the attempt to overcome disadvantage without denying difference.

How should this be achieved? The politics of difference perspective recognises the androcentricity of organisations and seeks to change it, thus facilitating women's full participation on equal terms. It is a longer-term strategy towards EO than either equal treatment, PA or PD, and recognises, and indeed celebrates, diversity. Mainstreaming policies are those which respect and respond to differences, rather than seeking to assist women to fit into male institutions and cultures by becoming 'more like men' (Cockburn 1991).

Many feminist writers have moved away from notions of equality and equal treatment to focus increasingly on the androcentricity of institutions and the superstructure (Smith 1987). The task is to challenge and change the male-streamism of organisations, illuminating how employers are not gender-neutral but, for example, privilege criteria for promotion (such as longevity of service and unbroken careers) which automatically and systematically favour one gender rather than the other. From this perspective, the trans-formation of institutions becomes the agenda, rather than the continuing attempt to improve women's access to and performance within organisations and their hierarchies as they are.

An example of the internationalisation of the male norm in thinking which is reflected in discourse and policy comes from the European Commission (EC) and its documentation on employment and employment policy. The term used in the EC to describe patterns of work for the most part undertaken by women (such as part-time and temporary employment) is 'atypical work' (see Chapter 4; McGiveney 1994; Meulders *et al.* 1994). The term itself indicates the idea that there is a male norm of working behaviour, which is adopted as a universal, from which many women deviate and against which they are measured. An agenda to transform would seek to normalise the plethora of working arrangements followed by many women and some men, rather than considering them in the context of deviation from a particular pattern followed by most men.

It is women's own experiences of unease or discomfort when seeking to fit in with the male norm which have prompted this approach. Italian feminist trade unionists, for example, have described how, in order to participate in 'masculine models of trade union militancy', they had to deny their femininity. To gain equality, they faced internal conflicts which they poignantly describe as '*lacerazione*' (lacerations). Becoming integrated entailed feeling 'mutilated' (Beccalli 1984: 201). They determined that it was better to change the unions, rather than changing themselves in order to seek equality within them. Parallel experiences have been reported by women who set up their own businesses, rather than work as employees in male dominated work cultures which they find alien-ating (Muir 1997; Rees 1992b, chapter 9). Similarly, there are studies of women in male dominated jobs who report they have to behave 'like a man' as a survival strategy (Breakwell 1985) and of able senior women managers who drop out mid-career from the stress of gender dissonance (Marshall 1995; Tanton 1994). There are also accounts of what women's education could and should be like (Coats 1994), and views from women students who are angry about what they see as the masculinist culture of their education and training organisations and who seek alternative styles of provi-sion (Taking Liberties Collective 1989).

But how feasible is it to introduce the concept of diversity into an organisation or, indeed, into training policy? How possible is it to change the value put on activities which are gendered? The next section looks at approaches to integrating models of EO, including mainstreaming, into training policies.

EO POLICIES IN TRAINING: TINKERING, TAILORING, TRANSFORMING

These three conceptualisations of EO (equal treatment, PA and PD, and mainstreaming equality) can be linked to three approaches to EO in education and training policy: I have called them 'tinkering', 'tailoring' and 'transforming' (Rees 1994a, 1995b, 1995c).[5]

Tinkering

Tinkering is essentially about 'tidying up' the legislation and procedures for equal treatment. This includes providing a sound legal base with adequate resources to ensure law enforcement. While limited in its effectiveness, the law nevertheless has some capacity to change practice and policy. In the UK, recent legislation on disability and on the Welsh language has prompted considerable interest in and development of policies to deliver equal treatment on these two equality dimensions on the part of employers whose activities are covered by the law.

The next step is formulating a policy on EO and incorporating a clear commitment to it in all documentation and procedures. Procedures include the introduction of gender monitoring devices and reporting mechanisms, training in EO awareness raising for staff, and paying attention to EO in evaluation and reporting procedures. This enables education and training providers and funders to measure performance in relation to equal access more effectively, to make adaptations to practice where appropriate, and to give out a clear message of intent on EO to all concerned.

However, as West and Lyon (1995: 60, drawing on Jewson and Mason 1986: 317) have pointed out:

> the existence of a formal policy can be, at the very least, an excuse for complacency. Management, having instituted change, especially when under pressure to do so, seems particularly prone to a conviction that equal opportunity 'now exists'.

The commitment to a policy certainly is not always accompanied by even the minimal proposed requirements of tinkering to ensure that it is delivered. Organisations which claim that they are 'moving towards becoming an EO employer', rather than claiming to be one already, show some degree of understanding of the complexities.

At the very least, gender monitoring is required to measure performance. Many organisations, especially in the public sector, now collect information on ethnic origin and disability of applicants as part of monitoring mechanisms in special sheets detached from the general application forms passed on to selectors. However, data on gender and age are more difficult to disguise in an application form or curriculum vitae. Nevertheless, gender monitoring has proved a useful tool in alerting education and training providers to the significance of gender as an organising principle in the allocation of staff to positions (by subject and level), and of students and trainees to courses and subjects. Financial analyses can be used to compare the allocation of expenditures by gender.[6]

Efforts aimed at awareness raising and training on issues of EO expanded considerably in many large organisations during the 1990s. Some (for example Queen's University, Belfast) used a cascade model of training, where employees who were participants in an initial first round of training sessions on EO are then used to provide training for others. This is clearly cheaper than hiring external trainers to train the entire workforce, but its impact depends crucially on the level of understanding, commitment and ability of the trainees-turned-trainers. Moreover, such exercises can prove counter-productive. Busy people are quick to judge and to withdraw from what they see as diversions from their everyday work commitments for training that they do not regard as necessary and important in the first place, especially if it fails to engage or convince them.

Awareness raising is essential but it needs to be convincing. In addition to setting clear objectives and designing criteria upon which progress can be assessed, it is clearly necessary to incorporate monitoring, evaluation and reporting procedures on EO to measure progress achieved and identify obstacles to the further development of EO. Building EO objectives into the responsibilities of all staff can be effective: if employees are asked as part of their annual performance reviews what they have done to facilitate EO, and to check on the performance of others in this regard, this can have a dramatic effect on the desire to understand and develop effective EO measures.

'Tinkering', then, is a minimum requirement for a learning organisation to move towards being an EO employer. Political arithmetic can be a powerful tool in revealing the impact of characteristics such as gender, race and age in the allocation of positions and opportunities to train or to study, even when equal treatment apparently offers no legitimate obstacles to individuals or groups. To 'not know' how the organisation performs on such criteria is not an adequate response, as Boddy (1995) points out with respect to TECs' performance on the part of their contracts regarding EO for members of ethnic minorities. However, although tinkering is necessary, it is not a sufficient measure to bring about EO.

Tailoring

Tailoring (PA and PD) involves the use of supplementary and support measures and sanctions to encourage more effective equality of access. It allows for 'add-on', supplementary measures to take account of women's 'special' position: 'nips and tucks' to accommodate their different shape. It might include initiatives to pre-train women in areas where they are under-represented and where there is a shortage of skills, for example in new technologies or management. Women-only training, women role models and tutors, earmarking of budgets for guidance and counselling, and documenting examples of good practice are common forms of tailoring (see Chapters 7 and 8).

Part of the reason why women are in a 'special position' compared with men lies in the fact that a substantial amount of their time is taken up with domestic commitments, and this restricts their opportunity to engage in training. Childcare provision or allowances and family-friendly hours can be regarded as 'tailoring' training provision to suit women. Given their 'special needs' due to their relative immobility, distance learning is a relatively under-explored but expanding form of training delivery (Curran 1995; Kirkup and von Prümmer 1997).

Tailoring can go further than this, however, by seeking to ensure that language, materials and illustrations in course documentation and guidance materials used in training are appropriate for women as well as men. Checks on the inclusiveness of all literature and course materials for both genders are important here. Some organisations 'gender-proof' their publications before releasing them; indeed, I have been asked to gender-proof several EC documents in recent years.

Women-only training workshops are a form of tailoring in that they, too, respond to women's 'special needs'. This form of provision proliferated in the 1980s and 1990s throughout the EU, partly because of financial support available from the European Social Fund. The IRIS network, funded by the EC Employment, Industrial Relations and Social Affairs Directorate-General (DGV) is made up of such women's training organisations throughout the EU (see Chapter 8). Significant strides forward have been made in introducing PA measures in training, partly prompted by demographic changes which made women returners a welcome alternative source of students. Lessons from woman-centred training pioneered in women-only training workshops outside mainstream provision, such as arranging contact hours to be family-friendly, the development of confidence building, and childcare needs being addressed, are to a limited extent being incorporated into the mainstream in courses geared for women returners.

However, positive action approaches are rooted in a focus upon inequalities of outcome and seek to address these through what can be described as a 'deficit model', that is, by focusing on the characteristics of the underperforming group and making good their 'deficiencies' (Bernstein 1971). Patterns of outcome are clearly important. But as Squires (1994) argues, theoretical discussions and policies about gender (and racial) injustice which are restricted to issues of EO shift the debate from oppression and domination back to the question of distribution. This, she maintains (1994: 1):

> leads away from analyses of structural systems of oppression to a debate of reallocation of resources or privileges to individuals, i.e., a narrowly distributive conception of justice.

This focus supports the structural *status quo* and diverts attention from the institutional framework, thus rendering it 'safe'. It is clearly essential, therefore, that EO policies move beyond such distributive concerns to more fundamental issues about the nature of the organisation and developing cultures which celebrate diversity while eliminating institutional disadvantage. This is the approach to EO in training I have described as transforming the mainstream.

Transforming

Transforming training provision builds upon the concept of politics of difference and seeks to 'feminise the mainstream' or mainstream equality. It implies moving beyond add-on policies to support and encourage women's participation. It involves a paradigm shift from the thousand flowers of good practice we know to be blooming from various compendia (CEEP, ETUC and UNICE 1995) and from specialist women's training projects (IRIS 1993) to mainstreaming good practice. This long-term strategy is designed to place women's training needs and the realities of their daily lives centre stage in the policy development of all education and training providers and in the design of all programmes through changing organisational cultures and institutions.

Transforming builds upon some of the foundations laid down in the shorter-term strategies, for example clear objectives, smooth running gender monitoring systems, and developed awareness and expertise throughout organisations at all levels. Rather than fitting women into existing structures and systems, or seeking to adjust structures to ensure a better fit, transforming involves designing programmes and projects informed by knowledge of the diversity of needs of potential participants. It includes the development of mission statements, aims and objectives, performance indicators and output measures. Evaluative studies should examine both quantitative and qualitative dimensions of women's training experiences. Particular attention should be paid to the development of a culture of EO awareness. EO audits where appropriate are necessary to support the transformation process and invoke sanctions.

As in any business objective, resources are required to implement transforming measures successfully. However, it should be added, the cost of *not* mainstreaming is rarely assessed (but see Breugal and Perrons 1995; Humphries and Rubery 1995). Indeed, some commentators have pointed to the improvements in the effectiveness of an organisation through employing a diverse workforce in the longer term (Kandola and Fullerton 1994; Ross and Schneider 1992).

The transforming agenda is predicated upon the argument that opportunities to participate in education, training and employment should not be enhanced or restricted by membership of one group or another. Legislation can be effective in ensuring a minimalist approach, but is highly restricted in its effects (Gregory 1987). The task in transforming, then, is to win hearts and minds, to recognise the complexities of EO and to build organisations, policies and projects informed by a desire to accommodate and benefit from the strengths of diversity. Building ownership of the EO agenda is clearly vital, while at the same time having all employees responsible for reporting on what progress they are making in achieving objectives helps to ensure action and attention move beyond rhetoric.

Cockburn demonstrated the ineffectiveness of some EO policies that are tacked on through her very valuable, detailed empirical study of four organisations which had sought to introduce them. She argues that there is a conflict between the short agenda of EO: 'the minimum position supported by management' and the long agenda 'involving more substantial kinds of change, the aim of equality activists, official and unofficial'. So, while management may be interested in removing 'the sex-biases from their human resource management practices' to widen the recruitment net for top jobs, this does not stretch as far as changing the culture of the organisation to make those women in senior positions feel comfortable. While some men at the top may be supportive of PA measures to accommodate women's domestic responsibilities, this is largely 'because they were increasingly aware of the imperative of competing for women's labour in a tightening labour market . . . '. However, the issue of valuing women's skills and labour ' . . . rarely makes it on to the management equality agenda' (all quotations from Cockburn 1991: 216/217). The long agenda (which I have called transforming, or mainstreaming) by contrast seeks to tackle deeply rooted organisational cultures and practices within which inequalities are embedded. It involves questioning the nature of the organisation and power relations within it; it means not simply looking at barriers to women's progress up the ladder, but asking whether the ladder is the right shape and size, or even whether it is necessary to have a ladder at all. In addition to standard EO practices which seek to monitor participation by gender and provide facilities such as childcare to accommodate domestic responsibilities (Moss 1990b), transforming addresses the gendered nature of the curriculum and who determines it, the values embodied in the organisation, the reproduction of its culture, the issues of cost-effectiveness and evaluation, and the allocation of resources.

While there is a detectable change in discourse from EO to 'managing diversity' in management 'how-to' books and among management gurus, as Kandola and Fullerton (1994) describe, the two approaches are quite different, the latter being much wider in its remit. There are, however, many different views among employers as to what managing diversity entails (Liff 1996), and, as yet, relatively little empirically grounded research.

The meeting point between managing diversity and transforming or mainstreaming equality is, of course, that both potentially move beyond the narrow definition of EO in terms of gender and include other dimensions of inequality such as race, sexual orientation and disability. The scope of the EC to address discrimination in terms of race is limited because of the retention of sovereignty on the issue of citizenship by Member States (see Chapter 5), although there are training projects for 'migrant' and ethnic minority groups. There has been little attention paid to the issue of sexual orientation in EC measures despite British evidence that many gay men and women fear coming out at their place of work, and those who do come out experience discrimination (Snape *et al.* 1995). At the EU level, disability remains an issue for 'special treatment' such as the HELIOS and HORIZON strand of DGV's EMPLOYMENT Community Initiative (see Chapter 8).

CONCLUSION

This chapter has sought to deconstruct some of the competing versions of the concept of EO. It has drawn distinctions between the models which underlie equal treatment, positive action and positive discrimination and mainstreaming equality approaches, and identified policy implications for each in the field of training. While many employers and education and training providers would regard themselves as EO employers, and have introduced practices rooted in an equal treatment model, the evidence on outcome, in terms of segregation by subject and occupation, indicates the limitations of such an approach. While there are some excellent examples of positive action training projects, they tend to depend upon piecemeal funding and to be outside mainstream training provision. Introducing policies designed to mainstream equality would require a radical overhaul of praxis and philosophy. The work on this has hardly begun.

Chapter 4

The European Union and equal opportunities

Europe has done a great deal for women. We like to remind everyone of the essential role as a driving force that the Commission has played with regard to equality, and the considerable legislative groundwork for important changes in attitudes, in the practices on [*sic*] the labour market and in the development of women's individual rights. But if it can be said that Europe has done much for women, it can also be said that women have done much for Europe.

(Jacques Santer, President of the European Commission, speaking at the 1995 International Women's Day conference organised by DGIX's Equal Opportunities Unit (CEC 1995b: 1))

On taking up office as President of the European Union in 1995, Jacques Santer was faced with a plethora of new Commissioners seeking the equality portfolio. Up until then it had been exclusively part of the duties of Commissioner Padraig Flynn, who was responsible for the Directorate-General (DG) for Employment and Social Affairs (DGV) and Education, Training and Youth (DGXXII, newly upgraded from being a Task Force). Commissioner Flynn, whose record on EO was controversial[1] was faced with competition from new Commissioners Edith Cresson from France, Monica Wulf-Matheis from Luxembourg, Anita Gradin from Sweden and Erkki Liikanen from Finland. There are as a consequence now five Commissioners who share responsibility for this area of work and who sit on a committee chaired by the President.

One of the first initiatives taken by President Jacques Santer on behalf of the committee was to write to all the Directors General of the Commission to ask them what was being done to further EO within their DGs. The responses to this were most instructive. While some documented internal and external activities, others interpreted the task solely in terms of in-house policies aimed at bringing about

EO for Commission staff within the DG.[2] A few DGs, however, responded that the issue of EO was not one that was directly relevant to their work. This gives an indication of the range of views among the most senior of the Commission's civil servants as to the significance of EO for their work.

Historically, it is frequently argued, the European Union and the Economic European Community before it acted as a catalyst to the development of equal opportunities in its Member States (Rossilli 1997). Women in Italy, Ireland and Greece in particular are regarded as having benefited from this influence as the European law, for example on equal pay, was more advanced than what was in place within those Member States (Roelofs 1995). The same policies have been criticised, however, for weakness of direction and implementation (Duncan 1996), for applying 'men's rules for women's rights' (Hoskyns 1992: 22), for having very little impact on broad patterns of gender segregation in the labour market (Mazey 1988; Roelofs 1995; Warner 1984) and for leading to a 'levelling down' of EO in some areas (Duncan 1996; Hoskyns and Luckhaus 1989; Rossilli 1997).

Although the Article in the Treaty of Rome relating to equal treatment of men and women on the issue of pay appeared to be largely ignored by the Member States in the late 1950s and 1960s, it was followed up by a series of hard and soft legislative measures and positive action initiatives which ensured at least some impact in the 1970s. More recent Directives on part-time work and pregnancy demonstrate a recognition of the implications of differences between men and women for equal treatment in the labour force. The recent accession of Sweden and Finland, which have a gender contract where women are viewed more as individuals rather than homemakers, adds expertise and experience of EO to the EU beyond that of most of the more long-standing members. Current debates on EO in the EC focus on the issue of mainstreaming, although there are many competing ideas of what such a concept entails (discussed in Chapter 10).

There has been some progress, then, in both conceptual and legislative terms on EO. In addition to the actions of the EU, the European Court of Justice (ECJ) has been widely recognised as having a significant role in the furtherance of EO through its liberal interpretation of the law in a series of crucial test cases. Many Member States have been successfully prosecuted for failing to adhere to European law on EO through the ECJ.

This chapter summarises and then critiques EO developments in the EU to the present day, with a special emphasis on its actions on training and labour market issues. It begins by outlining the legislative progress and the impact of the ECJ. It then traces the shift in the EC approach to EO through the models set out in Chapter 3, from equal treatment to positive action to contemporary concerns about 'mainstreaming' equality measures. The complexity of EO as a policy objective and the limitations of the competence and effectiveness of the EC are underlined by the failure of measures so far to provide much more than a legislative framework, some awareness-raising through the development of networks, and examples of funded positive action projects representing 'good practice' in a variety of fields. Equal pay between men and women, the focus of much of the attention so far, is far from being achieved. Gender segregation, both in training (Rees 1995a) and in the workforce (Rubery and Fagan 1993), as we saw in Chapter 2, remains very marked. And, as yet, there has been little progress on extending the concern for EO beyond gender to include other dimensions of inequality.

EQUAL TREATMENT LEGISLATION

As part of its strategy to seek constant improvement in living and working conditions, and to ensure fair conditions for competition, the EEC enshrined the principle of equal pay for men and women in Article 119 of the Treaty of Rome in 1957. This was particularly pushed for by France which feared unfair competitive advantage accruing to other Member States through the use of a low-paid female workforce: at the time France was the only founder Member State which had begun to address this issue in its own national legislative framework (van Overbeek 1994). The move was fuelled also by the concept of equality for all citizens in the aftermath of the Second World War (Meehan 1993). These concerns took precedence over any particular gender equality agenda. Conceived in the context of a purely economic European Community, Article 119 states that Member States must ensure and maintain the principle that men and women receive equal pay for equal work.

However, there was no implementation of Article 119 in the Member States, and it was clear that legislation at the national level would be needed to make it effective. Hence, despite some opposition, the commitment to equal pay expressed in the Treaty of Rome was followed up by a series of Directives passed in the 1970s on equal pay for work of equal value, equal treatment for men and women as regards access to employment, vocational training and promotion, working conditions, and social security (see Table 4.1). It was perhaps during this period that the greatest headway was made on equal treatment, as all national governments introduced equality legislation in order to comply. In Ireland this meant a fundamental change in the status of married women in the labour force (Hoskyns 1988).

In 1982, a Commission Decision led to the setting up of an Advisory Committee on Equal Opportunities for Men and Women (82/43/EEC). More recently, Directives in the late 1980s and early 1990s have addressed the issues of equal treatment in occupational social security systems and extending coverage to the self-employed and people in family businesses who were omitted from the 1970s Directives. 'Wives' working in the agricultural sector in particular secured protection during pregnancy and motherhood, and gained access to pensions in their own right. Safety and health at work of pregnant workers, and workers who have recently given birth or who are breastfeeding, are also addressed. These latter Directives can be seen in the spirit of needing to address some of the differences between men and women which need to be accommodated in order to tender them 'equal treatment' (Hoskyns 1996).

These Directives have whittled away some of the more glaring

Table 4.1. The EC equality Directives

1975	On equal pay for work of equal value (75/117)
1976	On equal treatment in access to employment, vocational training, promotion, and working conditions (76/207)
1978	On equal treatment in social security matters (statutory social security schemes) (79/7)
1986	On equal treatment in occupational social security schemes (86/378)
1986	On equal treatment of the self-employed (including spouses working in family businesses) including in the agricultural sector, and on the protection of self-employed women during pregnancy and motherhood (86/613)
1992	On the introduction of measures to encourage improvements in the safety and health at work of pregnant workers, workers who have recently given birth, or are breastfeeding (92/85)

inequalities in pay and social security between men and women, including family workers, and those caused as a result of pregnancy. Their significance lies in the clarification of the Treaty of Rome; for example, the 1975 Equal Pay Directive made it clear that 'pay' includes sick pay and occupational pensions, and that collective bargaining can be used in addition to individuals bringing cases. To an extent, this has moved the focus away from discrimination based on the characteristics of a complainant to tackling the more subtle issue of discrimination rooted in generalised assumptions about categories of people: hence the significance of the 1976 Equal Treatment Directive is that it introduced the important principle of indirect discrimination (discussed in Chapter 3). This is where there is unequal treatment on the grounds of characteristics other than sex but whereby, nevertheless, people of one sex are disadvantaged. It is immaterial whether or not there is any intention to discriminate.

Directives are binding and take precedence over national law. However, Member States have discretion as to how to achieve the desired results. They have a duty to amend laws, regulations and administrative provisions which are contrary to Directives. There are variations, however, in the extent to which Member States implement them, in some cases because of constitutional problems (see below). Also, there are many gaps yet to be filled, for example those caused by the vexed issue of the relationship between pensionable age and retirement age – an issue of particular pertinence in the UK. Finally, it is alas the case that the approach taken to bringing about equal treatment has not always been to extend the rights of men to women: in a number of instances, such as retirement age and social security, Member States have 'levelled down', for example by closing the gender gap by raising women's retirement age to that of men rather than vice versa. In other instances where what was required by national law was better than the standard introduced by European law, Member States have again taken the opportunity to level down (Hoskyns and Luckhaus 1989; Rossilli 1997).

Two new Directives, at the planning stage for many years, have been persistently blocked by the Social Affairs Council of Ministers: these focus upon parental leave and the reversal of the burden of proof. In cases of equal pay, the latter would mean that the employer would have to prove that the principle of equality had not been violated rather than the plaintiff needing to prove that discrimination had taken place. Other proposed Directives which would be of significance to women in the labour market focus on part-time and temporary work (see Prechal *et al.* 1994).

Another new proposal, to amend Directive 86/378 on equal treatment for men and women in occupational social security schemes to bring it into line with case law following the Barber judgement of 17 May 1990 and subsequent judgements, is more likely to succeed. This will acknowledge that all forms of benefit derived from employees' occupational social security schemes constitute an element of 'pay' within the meaning of Article 119 of the Treaty of Rome. The original Directive allowed for certain 'derogation' (or deviation) from the principle of equal treatment, for example on retirement age and survivors' benefits (EC 1995b). The proposed amendment is currently going thorough the process of approval by being considered by the European Parliament, the Economic and Social Committee and the Council of Ministers.

Resolutions and recommendations

Some of the follow-up EO legislation proposed by the EC has taken the form of Community 'soft law', in other words Council Resolutions and Commission Recommendations.[3] These are not legally binding. There is, of course, even wider variation between Member States in the extent to which soft law is implemented than there is on 'hard law'. Like the later Directives on EO, these Resolutions and Recommendations move beyond the *laissez faire*, equal treatment approach, and are based on a recognition of the differences between men and women. They are designed to address some of the disadvantages women experience in the labour market through positive action measures. Recommendations and Resolutions on EO of particular relevance are set out in Table 4.2.

The 1984 *Recommendation on the Promotion of Positive Action for Women* is of especial significance here, as it entailed the adoption of a positive action policy within the framework of national policies and practices aimed at 'eliminating' inequalities affecting women in working life and promoting a better balance between the sexes in employment. Similarly, the 1987 *Recommendation on Vocational Training for Women* and the series of Council Resolutions on the promotion of EO in Structural Funds created an opportunity for positive action measures in the field of training. These are discussed in Chapters 7 and 8.

Table 4.2.   Selected Recommendations and Resolutions on equal
treatment of men and women

1982	Retirement age (82/357)
1984	The promotion of positive action for women (84/331)
1984	On combating unemployment among women (84/161)
1987	On vocational training for women (87/342)
1990	On the protection of the dignity of women and men at work (90/157)
1992	On sexual harassment and the protection of dignity of men and women at work (92/31)
1992	On childcare and parental leave (92/241)
1994	On the promotion of equal opportunities for men and women through action by the European Structural Funds (94/231)
1994	On equal participation by women in an employment-intensive economic strategy within the EU (94/368)
1995	On the balanced participation of men and women in decision-making (95/168)

European Court of Justice[4]

The ECJ has surprised many commentators by its liberal approach to legislation on EO. It has prosecuted individual Member States and brought them into line. It has found in favour of individual women bringing cases against employers or Member States. It has facilitated further strengthening of EO through case law. Nevertheless, it has made clear that it is not in the business of altering relationships between the genders in family relationships: inequalities in power and domestic duties remain unchallenged by the ECJ. This is, of course, a major weakness in its effectiveness as a change agent in EO as the nature of the gender contract within Member States remains intact.

There are numerous authoritative accounts of the work of the ECJ generally and with respect to EO specifically (see Hoskyns 1996 for the most recent detailed analysis). This section identifies a few of the cases, in chronological order, which illustrate an underlying model of EO, drawing attention to the contribution and limitation of the ECJ in acting as a catalyst to a more sophisticated understanding and delivery of EO policies.

Gabrielle Defrenne, an air hostess with Sabena, the Belgian State airline, brought the first EO cases to the ECJ in the 1970s, which included the claim that she was being paid less than a man whose job title was different but whose work was the same (Case 43/75). The Belgian national court, to which she originally brought the cases, was unsure whether Article 119 could be relied upon by private individuals to secure their rights in the Treaty of Rome, and so it requested the ECJ to make a ruling. While she lost her cases on severance pay, pensions and retirement age, the ECJ awarded her the equal pay case. In the judgement, the importance of equality between men and women as a general principle of Community law was underlined by the Court and attention was drawn to the responsibility of all institutions (including national courts) to see that it is upheld. This case was highly significant, in that the decision made clear that Article 119 could be used by private individuals in national courts.

In the Rinner–Kuhn case (Case 171/88), the ECJ ruled against a German employer who had used German law to avoid making sickness payments to an employee who had worked less than ten hours a week. Similarly, in a case where a local authority was refusing a severance grant on retirement to part-time staff (Kowalska, Case 33/89), it ruled that different treatment of part-time workers has to be justified by the employer. As the vast majority of part-time workers in the EU are women, the ECJ ruled that treating part-time workers differently from full-time workers represents indirect discrimination against women. This was a significant step in the recognition of the concept of indirect discrimination. Nevertheless, despite these judgements, discrimination against part-time workers remains a significant problem (Prechal and Senden 1994).

Probably the most well known EO cases to come before the ECJ are the three Ds: Danfoss, Dekker and Dansk. In the Danfoss case (Case 109/88), the ECJ placed the obligation on the employer to show that difference in treatment of employees was not based on their sex. This foreshadowed the proposed, but so far ill-fated, Directive aimed at reversing the burden of proof. Rulings in the cases of Dekker (Case 177/88) and Dansk (Case 178/88) established that dismissal on the grounds of pregnancy represents direct discrimination and hence contravenes the Equal Treatment Directive. More recently, the ECJ made a far-reaching judgement that part-time workers should be given the same rights as full-time workers. This has particular implications in those Member States such as the UK where rates of part-time work among women are high. However, some momentum was lost when a case contesting positive action for women was successfully brought before the ECJ in 1995 (see below).

The ECJ, then, has contributed to conceptualisations of EO and, by addressing the issue of part-time workers and pregnancy, has moved from equal treatment to the acknowledgement of group differences between men and women. However, it has avoided other issues relating to the imbalance between men and women in terms of domestic responsibilities which lie at the heart of much of the difference in outcome in education, training and the labour market. Hoskyns argues that, by emphasising employment rights over social security, the Court has in effect limited its own jurisdiction by 'tipping the policy in a certain direction' (Hoskyns 1996: 162). The European Network of Women, a lobby group of some significance made up of various grass-roots women's organisations, has been putting pressure on policymakers to develop a more diverse programme (Pillinger 1992). This would need to be one that recognises that much of the poverty of opportunity experienced by women is rooted in the restrictions on their freedom to participate in education, training and the labour market at all. Equal treatment within these arenas is inevitably restricted in its effectiveness at combating this gross form of inequality.

The Commission, as the Community's 'watchdog' (van Overbeek 1994: 30), has initiated a number of infringement procedures against Member States identified as defaulting on equal treatment law (see Pillinger 1992: Appendix 4, for examples based on the 1975 Equal Pay Directive). One taken against the UK eventually led to the Equal Pay for Work of Equal Value (1984) amendment to the Equal Pay Act (1970) legislation being passed to bring UK law into line with the Directive. Private plaintiffs have also contributed by bringing cases to their national courts when Member States have not fully implemented the provisions of Directives into national laws. The ECJ has itself required national courts to interpret their national legislation in accordance with the content of Directives. This has provided cover in situations where private individuals could not invoke the law, for example against other private individuals.

Of course, the extent to which Member States implement the European legislation varies considerably, and the provisions of the various Member States' own legal systems have varying strengths and weaknesses. While the UK has a reasonably good record on implementing EU legislation (that it has not vetoed), regional assemblies in Italy may resist implementing laws agreed to on their behalf by the nation state in fields where they have competence. This issue of variable practice in implementation means that it is most unwise to read off practice from legal provision. Nevertheless, Collins (1992: 107) points to variation in legal provision between Member States by citing the following examples of good practice which could be emulated:

> the Italian law which states that the employees of a sub-contractor must receive wages as high as those of primary employees; the German law which gives all home-workers the full status of employees; and the French statutory minimum-wage system.

Equal treatment legislation in the Member States is well docu-mented (see van Overbeek 1994), and reviewed regularly by the EC's *Network of Experts on the Implementation of the Equality Directives.* The most recent review reports slow progress. While more severe sanctions are being imposed in cases of breach of the equality principle in the UK and Denmark than in other Member States, Prechal and Senden (1994: 61) conclude that, at the other end of the continuum, 'German legislation . . . is giving cause for concern as it appears to be resulting in serious backward steps.' The reunification of Germany, *inter alia*, has meant addressing the fact that very different sets of legislation and provision for women had prevailed in the German Democratic Republic and the Federal Republic of Germany. In effect the breadwinner/homemaker gender contract of the Federal Republic is now being imposed on women of the new Länder through the law, with deleterious effects for their rights.

Prechal and Senden's (1994) words proved to be somewhat prophetic, as it was a plaintiff from Germany who subsequently used the equal treatment legislation to bring a case to the ECJ over the use of employment quotas as a positive action measure to increase the proportion of women working in the City of Bremen Parks Department. The Court ruled that the use of such quotas was incompatible with the 1976 Equal Treatment Directive. The City of Bremen was interpreted as having gone 'too far' in its policy by guaranteeing women priority: positive action was intended only to promote EO. As Elaine Vogel-Polsky commented:

> the question is whether the right of each individual not to be

discriminated against on grounds of sex, a right which has been recognised by the Court as a fundamental right, should take precedence over the rights of a disadvantaged group, in this case women, to be compensated for past (and current) discrimination?

(Vogel-Polsky, quoted in EC 1996c: 4)

After considerable debate and consultation with legal experts, in this case the Court came down on the side of a very literal interpretation of the law. The case may well set back progress on positive discrimination to redress past discrimination and disadvantage.

Nielson and Szyszczak (1991: 82) argue that it has taken individual litigation to 'breathe life' into the equal pay principle. However, as studies of those who have brought equal pay and sex discrimination cases in the UK courts have shown (Leonard 1987b), such struggles need considerable commitment and support from trade unions and the EOC, and success is unlikely. Indeed, only a fraction of those who embark on the road to court ever reach it, and fewer still achieve a satisfactory outcome. Nevertheless the ECJ has provided an opportunity for individual litigants to pursue cases with some success, and the case law that has developed has been an important contribution to the development of EO in the EU.

POSITIVE ACTION: THE FIRST AND SECOND MEDIUM TERM ACTION PROGRAMMES ON EO

Clearly, simply legislating that there should be equal treatment of men and women was always likely to be limited in its effects. In 1976, the EC set up an Equal Opportunities Unit, in Directorate General V, Employment, Industrial Relations and Social Affairs (DGV) to monitor how existing equality legislation worked in practice and to draft new legislation for consideration by Ministers (including most of the Directives, Recommendations and Resolutions referred to above, together with a series of Proposals to Council). It was during the 1970s that much of the progress was made in this regard.

A Council Decision led to the setting up, in 1981, of an Advisory Committee on Equal Opportunities for Women and Men made up of national experts, which works closely with the Equal Opportunities Unit. The Committee tends to comprise representatives from the Member States working in the equality field and advises the EC on drafting EO policies. Originally it was intended simply to be a resource to the Commission, but, according to the Deputy Chair, during the late 1980s the Advisory Committee became more pro-active, taking some initiatives and seeking to move the equality agenda along more quickly (Boddendijk 1991).

The Equal Opportunities Unit, with the support of the Advisory Committee, developed measures to supplement the effects of the equality legislation in the form of a series of Medium Term Community Action Programmes. The first two Action Programmes were described as having the effect of raising the profile of EO throughout the Community (see CEC 1991a). The First Community Action Programme on the Promotion of Equal Opportunities for Women and Men (1982–5) aimed to 'strengthen the rights of the individual as a way of achieving equality and to bring about equal treatment' (Cunningham 1992: 180). This was to be achieved largely through positive action measures. This clearly represented a shift in policy whereby, in order to achieve equal treatment, it was deemed necessary to address the 'special' situation of women in the labour market.

The DGV Action Programme in fact focused on two main themes: the strengthening of individual rights through legal intervention; and the promotion of EO in practice by the use of positive action strategies. The first was tackled through the positive action 'soft law' enacted during this period (described earlier). To address the latter, a number of networks of independent experts in the Member States were set up by the Equal Opportunities Unit to support its activities. The networks were intended to facilitate cross-national learning, to develop contacts, to exchange information and experience on issues of importance to women, and to develop awareness. They worked with the EC on research and drafting EO programmes. The full list of equality networks is set out in Table 4.3.

The network on the position of 'women on [sic] the labour market' is largely research driven, and analyses obstacles facing women in employment and the balance between work and family life. Recent work has focused on atypical work and the impact of the Single Market on women in the textile and banking sectors. The local employment initiatives network's budget is used to support women who want to start up in business: some 400 women's local enterprise initiatives were approved for financial assistance in 1993 (Breakthrough 1994: 22). It also develops awareness-raising among local enterprises, for example in export possibilities.

The later networks listed were established during the Second

Table 4.3. The EC equality networks

1982	Application of equality directives
1982–3	Women on the labour market
1984	Local employment initiatives for women
1986	Positive action in enterprises
1986	Equal opportunities in broadcasting
1986	Childcare
1986	Equal opportunities in education
1988	IRIS – Women's training projects
1990	Women in decision making
1995	Families and work

Medium Term Community Action Programme (1986–90). This was set up in recognition of the limitations of the earlier Programme, and was more oriented towards prompting cooperation at Community level in specific actions geared towards target groups, such as single parents. It focused on seven central themes: law, education and training, employment, new technologies, social security, family responsibilities and consciousness-raising.

Attention was drawn to the specific need for EO in the field of training policy by the Recommendation on Vocational Training for Women in 1987. This called upon Member States to ensure that women have equal access to all types and levels of vocational training, particularly those professions likely to expand in the future, and those in which women have been historically under-represented (CEC 1987b). It also asked Member States to develop a range of measures: for example, to encourage awareness-raising and information dissemination, to sponsor spouses of the self-employed who help with the business, to support women setting up in business or returning to work, and to introduce supplementary measures such as childcare. This led to the setting up of the IRIS network of vocational training schemes for women and facilitated the funding of women's training projects through previous Community Action Programmes on education and training (discussed in Chapter 7) and the European Social Fund and LEONARDO DA VINCI, the EC's current Community Action Programme on training (discussed in Chapter 8).

The IRIS network was set up to increase good-quality training for women and raise the profile of women's training needs. It promotes exchanges, organises seminars, runs a database and produces publications on matters of relevance to those interested in women and training. IRIS has been regarded as highly effective in identifying training issues for women, and developing and documenting examples of good practice (PA Cambridge Economic Consultants 1992). It has also, through its bulletins, been an effective disseminator of policy development in Brussels on issues germane to women and training. In 1995, the network, which is run by the Centre for Research on Women (CREW), a women's cooperative, became independent of the EC (see Chapter 8).

The Advisory Committee on Equal Opportunities for Women and Men has consistently underlined the importance of women's training, both for the economy, and as a route to financial independence for women, thus avoiding social exclusion. The Women's Committee of the European Parliament and the European Women's Lobby (EWL) have been highly influential and have repeatedly stressed the importance of women's training. It is largely through their efforts that the Medium Term Action Programmes were set up.

Both the first and second Medium Term Action Programmes can be conceptualised as positive action measures. They established a framework within which Community legislation could be enacted, projects could be funded, the flow of information through networks could be facilitated, and the progress of EO could be monitored, all in recognition of aspects of the position of women in the labour market. The focus of the Third (1991–1995) and Fourth (1996–2000) Community Action Programmes on Equal Opportunities, however, moved to integration and mainstreaming in the context of the completion of the internal market. They can be read as a further paradigm shift in EC thinking towards EO.

MAINSTREAMING? THE THIRD AND FOURTH MEDIUM TERM ACTION PROGRAMMES ON EO

The main aim of the Third Community Action Programme on Equal Opportunities was to 'entrench equality policy as an integral part of the Community's economic and structural policies, and to promote women's full participation in economic and social life' (Cox 1993: 56). It can be seen as going further than earlier programmes in its analysis of what policies are needed to be effective. The objectives were to facilitate women's integration into the labour market, to reconcile employment and domestic responsibilities for women, and to improve the status of women in society

(CEC 1991a). One of the lessons from the earlier Programmes was that there was a need for more effective integration of the equality objective into all relevant policy areas: this is sought in the new phase.

The argument was made that 'Equal opportunities policy must not be treated as a separate policy but as an integral part of other policies, underpinning their effectiveness' (CEC 1991a: 86). However, it is clear that, even in this conceptualisation, the 'problem' is still identified, to an extent at least, as being women themselves: 'the idea is . . . to use legal instruments and an information and awareness campaign to *make them realise* just what their rights and opportunities are' (CEC 1991a: 7; my emphasis).

The Third Action Programme took place in the context of the completion of the Single Market and the Maastricht Treaty. A major theme of both is the development of human resources to create employment. The Maastricht Treaty incorporates the Community Charter of Fundamental Social Rights of Workers which includes an Article stating that every worker must have access to vocational training throughout their working life. Public authorities and the two sides of industry, it states, should set up continuing and permanent training systems enabling people to retrain where necessary. The Charter also includes an article on equal treatment for men and women which covers access to employment, pay, education and training, career development, working conditions and social protection. It specifically mentions that measures should be developed enabling men and women to reconcile their work and family responsibilities. This is a major theme of the Third Action Programme. The UK's opt-out of (what has now become known as) the Social Chapter of the Maastricht Treaty does not exclude it from the legal provisions on equal treatment between men and women provided for under the Treaty of Rome.

At this stage of the history of the EU, economic arguments for the development of women's skills were beginning to be regarded as highly significant in the overall economic policy aimed at creating a skilled workforce. The focus on developing human resources highlighted in the White Paper on economic policy, *Growth, Competitiveness and Employment* (EC 1994a), inevitably threw the spotlight on women, given that it is they who are the majority of the economically inactive and the unskilled. It is no surprise to find in the Third Programme, then, a more highly concerted effort on EO, with a particular focus on the integration of women into the labour market, and indeed, on the integration of EO into mainstream policy.

Improving legislative provisions remained a key part of activities under the Third Action Programme; the Directives and 'soft law' enacted during this period were outlined earlier in this chapter. EC monitoring activity was strengthened, and further clarification and guidelines on the implementation of the law produced. The main action proposed for tackling the objective of integrating women into the labour market was the Community Initiative known as the New Opportunities for Women (NOW) programme. This was set up in 1990 for five years and provided funds to Member States to promote vocational training and employment for women (especially the long-term unemployed and those who want to set up their own businesses). Operating under the Structural Funds, the resources made available for NOW have been limited, an estimated 120 mecus from the European Social Funds, European Regional Development Fund (ERDF) and co-financing from Member States, according to Nielson and Szyszczak (1991). Nevertheless, they mark a symbolic move towards integration (see Chapter 8). Funds were made available under the framework of transnational operations for co-financing action aiming to help women with their own enterprise development or to reintegrate then into the labour market. Supplementary measures were available for supporting childcare and providing technical assistance, particularly in the least-developed regions. Women have also benefited (as have men) from other Community Initiatives such as HORIZON, which is targeted at the disabled.

These Community Initiatives came to the end of their lives in 1995, when they were replaced by a single new human resources Community Initiative known as EMPLOYMENT, and made up of three strands: NOW, HORIZON and YOUTHSTART (the latter aimed at young people). Resources have been expanded considerably and the period for which the initiative is due to run has been doubled to ten years (see Chapter 8). Nearly half the projects in EMPLOY-MENT-NOW concern women setting up their own businesses. Others focus on aspects of gender segregation, both horizontal and vertical, and the development of methodologies for the creditation of women's skills (EC 1997; for an inventory of positive action in Europe see Serdjenian 1994). While many of these projects are likely to have a positive action approach, there are some examples of mainstreaming projects within EMPLOYMENT-NOW.

The issue of women's integration into the labour market was also tackled through a commitment to monitor participation in all co-financed Structural Fund projects (which take up a third of the EU financial commitments). This proved difficult to deliver (as Chapter 8 demonstrates). Other strategies to achieve integration lay in exhortation to Member States to integrate the equality dimension into their employment, educational and social policies, and to the Social Partners to incorporate EO policies into the collective bargaining process (CEC 1991b: 15,16). The Commission, using competence granted to it as defined under the Resolutions, committed itself to conducting further research and dissemination, fostering the exchange of information, publishing examples of good practice and enlarging the activities of various networks.

The objective of improving the status of women in society was mainly tackled through raising awareness and the dissemination of information. While some Commission Initiatives were taken in the field of women and the media, the EC considered that it was for the Member States 'to develop awareness of the need to portray female and male roles in a balanced way' (CEC 1991b: 21). The principles of subsidiarity and complementarity in Commission activities meant fine lines needed to be drawn to distinguish what were appropriate activities for the Commission to undertake to 'complement' those of the Member States. The emphasis was inevitably focused on transnational research and information-based activities. The Equal Opportunities Unit set up the network on women and decision-making during this period to try to encourage greater participation of women in all levels of decision-making processes.

Field (1995: 69) comments that:

> If the first three Action Programmes were relatively modest, the fourth Programme, for 1996 onwards, promises positive humility. Its most significant proposed content by mid-1995 was provision for an annual report on the situation of the Member States.

The annual report referred to (EC 1996f) turned out to be a fairly upbeat document which makes much of the potential of the main-streaming agenda of the Fourth Medium Term Action Programme on EO (1996–2000) and the Commissioners' group on EO between men and women mentioned at the beginning of this chapter. An interdepartmental group has been established to take this agenda forward. However, given the slipperiness of the concept, and the difficulties of instigating and delivering effective EO policies, this aim is clearly an ambitious one. Moreover, while the resources for NOW may have been increased, this needs to be put into the context of the fact that over half the funds at the disposal of the EU are spent on agriculture and fisheries: the budget available for the development of human resources as a whole is relatively modest, while the proportion of that budget spent on the equality agenda is minute.

The Fourth Medium Term Action Programme is more specific about its mainstreaming agenda, although it is too early to judge the results of this commitment. The Programme aims to promote the integration of EO into the preparation, implementation and monitoring of all EU and Member State activities, while being mindful of the sensitivities of culture within individual Member States – in effect, a subsidiarity get-out clause. It focuses on six key objectives: the exchange and development of information and experience of good practice, studies and research and the dissemination of information. The programme is managed by a Technical Assistance Office called ANIMA and a management committee. Again, the funds are modest, but there is the opportunity for a catalytic effect through the leverage of resources.

MOVING TOWARDS MAINSTREAMING?

The EC was one of the first major institutions to seek to ensure equal treatment for men and women on the grounds that, by treating individuals equally, discrimination will be removed. However, Article 119 (the legal basis), the six Directives, four Recommendations and four Action Programmes which have followed are still largely focused on equal pay and related labour market matters. There was some pressure on the Spring 1996 Intergovernmental Conference to revise the Treaty to broaden the scope of equal opportunities so as to include political, economic, social and cultural rights (CEC 1995b: 1), but not to much effect.

A number of serious criticisms can be levelled at the EC's approach to equal treatment. In the first instance, it is of course focused exclusively on equality between men and women. Inequalities between members of different racial and ethnic groups, between people of different sexual orientation, between the able-bodied and the disabled, between peoples of minority religious, linguistic and cultural groups, all remain unaffected for the most part by a legislative framework designed to address inequalities between the sexes. Measures for groups such as the disabled and ethnic minorities are still couched in a positive action model and tend to consist of small-scale initiatives or projects (see Chapter 8).

Second, there is the fundamental criticism that rights to equal treatment only apply to the citizens of the EU. The estimated thirteen million migrants who do not have citizen status include about eight million who are nationals of non-Member States, the majority of whom live in Germany (where there is a large Turkish population), France and the UK. Several commentators have pointed to the adverse effect that the strengthening of immigration control in the Single Market, together with deregulation measures designed to encourage employers to take on more workers, is likely to have on black and Asian people in particular (see, for example, Collins 1992).

Third, the majority of women (and indeed men) work for small and medium-size enterprises which are far more difficult than large employers to police on the implementation of equality legislation. Moreover, even with large employers, as Walby (1994/5) illustrates, strategies for developing EO in the workplace appear to be predicated upon more traditional Fordist modes of organisation: they are less successfully applied to the post-Fordist systems of zero-hours contracts, sub-contracting, flexible hours and temporary employment contracts which characterise the employment practices of an increasing proportion of employers (Lovering 1990).

Fourth, the legislation and action measures still rest upon a male model of employment. Equal treatment means equal to that afforded men; men are the starting point, the norm. This orientation is revealed in the wording used in the foreword of the EC's account of its role in developing EO for women and men, written by the (then) Director General of DGV, Jean Degimbe (1991: 6), which begins with the statement 'Women are men's equals'. The approach to EO is rooted in assumptions about how individuals engage with the labour market that are based upon 'normal' male patterns. These include assumptions governing the arrangements of pay, pensions and access to training which tend to be predicated upon the male pattern of lifelong membership of the labour force, whereas, for many women, membership is intermittent. Assumptions that workers expect lifetime earnings, mobility and, above all, full-time employment, inevitably mean not simply that there are gaps in the legislative provisions but that the starting point is inappropriate. The diversity of women's patterns are taken not as a given, to build upon, but as a peculiarity, a disadvantage. The use of the term 'atypical work' to describe the patterns of employment followed by millions of women and some men is perhaps the most obvious sign of the underlying androcentric thinking which has given rise to a severely limited legislative framework.

The superficially 'gender neutral' perspective is especially noticeable in relation to measures on social security and unemployment. The payment of lower pensions to women on the grounds that they tend to live longer than men is a nice example of how the male is taken as the starting point, although, as Nielson and Szyszczak (1991: 119) point out, increasingly as far as factors determining longevity are concerned: '[d]ifferences in social, occupational group, hereditary dispositions, smoking, alcohol and tobacco consumption may be more influential than a worker's sex'.

Fifth, it is clear that equal treatment is extremely problematic, given the different positions of men and women in the labour market and the home. The issue of gender contracts and their impact on women's ability to respond to 'equal opportunities' is not tackled, although there is more discussion of the balancing of home and work life and the position of women in decision-making. Rather than assisting some women to secure the same access as men to current rewards, it may be necessary to recognise that the politics of difference requires respecting a more diverse pattern of lives, allowing them to co-exist without incurring penalties for not conforming to a male norm. This entails facilitating more flexible arrangements for work, and for the care of children and the elderly. The emphasis in Directives on the rights of workers, rather than citizens, systematically disadvantages women. It is noticeable that the proposed Directives on parental leave (long opposed by the Conservative UK Government) and the reversal of the burden of proof, which would make a significant impact on women, have so far made tortuously slow progress through the approval stages, periodically grinding to a complete halt for years at a time.

Finally, the focus on integration still suggests that the onus is on women to change and fit in with the *status quo*: there is no suggestion of changing the patterns, values and priorities of the mainstream in order to accommodate a more diverse workforce. The concept of mainstreaming is expressed as one of integrating equality objectives into all policies. However, this may still leave the priorities, assumptions and values of the dominant culture untouched. Frank Boddendijk, Vice-Chair of the EC's Advisory

Committee on Equal Opportunities for Women and Men expresses a view of mainstreaming which comes far closer to one where the mainstream is transformed to accommodate diversity, rather than one where women are simply fitted in, or 'integrated':

> When we discuss the so-called women's question, we have to realise that it is not by definition women who constitute the problem. Why should an equal opportunities policy be directed at the integration of women into the existing system? Instead of integrating women into the system we need a transformation of the system, a transformation which responds to the needs and abilities of both women and men. A transformation . . . in short, which goes far beyond cosmetic changes and window dressing.
>
> (Boddendijk 1991: 96)

This issue of the difference between mainstreaming equality and transforming the mainstream is taken up and discussed further in later chapters.

CONCLUSION

The EC has taken action to seek to improve the position of women in the labour market in the EU. However, by basing such action on an equal treatment model that fails to take into account the effects of an uneven domestic division of labour, progress towards equality has necessarily been muted. Moreover, the complexities of EO mean that to impact upon the gendering of education, training and the labour market would require significantly more than legislation and positive action measures.

There are solid '*acquis*' or achievements. Legislation has been passed on the principle of equal treatment for men and women in access to equal pay, employment, vocational training and promotion, and in working conditions. The ECJ has consolidated those gains through case law. The Commission has acted as a catalyst in putting EO on the agenda in many of the EU Member States. Committees and networks have been set up and feed into the design of legislation and projects designed specifically for women. A considerable amount has been learnt about the causes of the rigidities of labour market segregation and the barriers to women's training. Nevertheless, underlying patterns of vertical and horizontal gender segregation in the labour market remain, and equal pay, the starting point for Article 119 in the Treaty of Rome, is far from being achieved. Gender segregation is at the same time both the cause of inequalities and the force inhibiting the effectiveness of EO policies. Clearly a more sophisticated understanding of the nature and causes of segregation is required, together with far more radical policies to reduce the impact of gender on occupational lifechances.

Chapter 5

Key issues in women's education and training in the UK

Q. Why do women never go to the moon?
A. Because it doesn't need cleaning.

Q. Why do women have small feet?
A. So they can get nearer the cooker.

Q. Why did the woman cross the road?
A. I have no idea. What was she doing out of the kitchen in the first place?

(Contemporary jokes in South Wales secondary schools)

Gender segregation characterises all known labour markets, although the degree of rigidity and the specificities of the patterns vary. Training systems play a significant role in underpinning such patterns of occupational segregation. This chapter draws out some key issues on women and post-compulsory education and training in the UK, a Member State of the European Union which, while similar to other members in many respects, differs significantly in others. It shares characteristics of skill shortages and the under-development and under-utilisation of women's skills. However, the UK is distinctive in that it has been particularly badly affected by the process of de-industrialisation and by the recession of 1991–94, it has a culture where both employers and employees seem reluctant to invest in training, and it has had a central government which has pursued policies of credentialism and marketisation of vocational education and training, which have had a distinct set of conse-quences.

Moreover, the labour force participation of women in the UK is characterised by a high proportion of women working part-time, the vast majority of whom have very little access to training and promotion opportunities. The UK is similar to Greece and Spain in that a high proportion of young people leave the education system at an early age compared with elsewhere (although staying-on rates are now increasing). It also has a relatively low level of provision of pre-school childcare compared with other EU Member States, despite having the third-highest proportion of women living as single parents. This clearly impacts upon women's capacity to participate in paid employment (Eurostat 1992).

The two issues which are the focus of this chapter cut across some of these similarities and differences. The first issue is the gendering of the discourse and organisation of education and training systems and the labour market to which they are linked. The second is gender as an organising principle in individuals' training trajectories and consequent patterns of participation in education and training systems. The extent to which institutions monitor and act upon those patterns of gender segregation is discussed. While these patterns of participation which characterise the UK training system are reflected to a greater or lesser degree elsewhere, the specificities in training culture and policy which set the UK apart from other Member States are explored.

The UK Conservative Government of the early to mid-1990s pursued a policy of the marketisation of public sector services (including training): this involved the shifting from state provision of public services towards a contract culture based on competition and 'quasi-markets' (Le Grand and Bartlett 1993). This is an approach which increasingly is influencing the policy development of some other Member States. Marketisation of training (Peck 1991), combined with the policy of creditation, the increasing attachment of formal qualifications to training, have had significant implications for the gendering of training and women's access to and participation in what is on offer.

The issue of the gendered nature of discourse is clearly germane to post-compulsory education and training in all Member States (even though the languages themselves are clearly quite different). And language is merely the outward and visible sign of a hegemony which determines the extent to which male and female students feel comfortable in different settings and courses, and the extent to which women teachers and trainers are able to compete successfully for senior positions in the hierarchies of education and training institutions and contribute to the construction of 'knowledge' which comes to characterise those subject areas. Feminist scholars of discourse have made considerable contributions to our understanding of the gendered significance of language (see Daly 1979), and attention is beginning to be focused on gendered meanings of the language of the workplace (Tannen 1995), if not as yet the training arena. The purpose of this section is to reconceptualise some of the key terms in the field of education, training and the labour market from a gendered perspective. Concepts such as skill, training, training systems and cultures, qualifications and career trajectories, all carry baggage as a consequence of their gendered social construction and warrant re-examination in the light of women's experiences. This section also examines the male hegemony of post-compulsory education and training: it discusses evidence of how the masculinist academic mode of production can alienate women and deter their participation as both consumers and providers.

It is in this context that the chapter then looks at patterns of gender segregation in post-compulsory education and training in the UK. This includes a 'political arithmetic' treatment of women's participation in training, in so far as statistics allow. The lack of systematic gender monitoring undertaken by training providers, and low levels of awareness of the potential significance of gender monitoring as a performance indicator, are shown here to compare badly with levels of awareness and availability of gender break-downs in statistics for education. Sources of data on participation in training in the UK have, however, recently been improved by the enhancement of the Labour Force Survey (LFS) and the new publi-cation series *Training Statistics* (see Employment Department 1995). Wales provides an interesting context here because it lies at one extreme of the UK in patterns of gender segregation in employ-ment, post-compulsory education and in training (Istance and Rees 1994). Once the region producing the highest proportions of both most and least qualified people, it now has the dubious distinction of having the highest proportion of school-leavers with no qualifi-cations, but no longer balancing this with large numbers of well qualified people. A range of policies is being introduced which seek to address the skills deficit in Wales (Welsh Office 1995). This extreme example throws some of the key issues in women and training in the UK into high relief.

Before discussing these themes in detail, however, it is important to stress that the UK differs from other Member States in two important regards with respect to EO which have a bearing on training matters. Despite the Sex Discrimination Act (which came into force in 1975), which prohibits discrimination on the grounds of gender in access to training, the UK is the only Member State which actively discriminates against some women's take-up of training opportunities on the grounds of their marital status (EOC 1993). Those unemployed married women in England and Wales who are ineligible for unemployment benefit, now known as the Job Seekers' Allowance (JSA), in their own right, are disallowed from participating in training programmes for the unemployed except at the discretion of local TECs. This is either on the grounds (for older women) that they have paid a reduced married woman's contribution to National Insurance, or that they are only available to work part-time. Similarly, while single parents may receive assistance with childcare while on such training programmes, married women may not (EOC 1993). This, combined with the lack of state-provided pre-school childcare, more generally sets the UK apart from other Members States where no such discrimination exists.

Second, the UK is the only Member State where most resident members of ethnic minorities have citizenship status and where a Race Relations Act (1976) legally prohibits discrimination on the grounds of race. In other Member States, many members of ethnic minorities are regarded as and called 'migrants', reflecting a second-class status with regard to citizens' rights. This can include restrictions on access to training. This is not to suggest of course that members of ethnic minorities in the UK enjoy equal access to and outcome from training provision: evidence on participation illustrates both indirect discrimination and structural barriers to participation (Boddy 1995).[1] Many positive action training programmes facilitated under the Act aimed at ethnic minorities are clearly cast in the deficit model (Bernstein 1971) and offer little in the way of transformative opportunities for skill enhancement that will significantly affect occupational lifechances. Nevertheless, the Act makes discrimination in the field of training on the grounds of race illegal and allows for some positive action provision. The lack of a legal infrastructure in other Member States and restrictions on mobility in the Single European Market for migrant workers leads to a legitimate concern among ethnic minorities in the UK about the worsening of conditions in 'Fortress Europe' (Mitchell and Russell 1994; Wrench and Solomos 1995).

The analysis of participation in training by ethnic minorities, like the identification and discussion of key issues in women's training in the UK, is seriously hampered by lack of research. Indeed, there is considerable imbalance in the UK research literature between the amount of attention paid to analyses of education, at all levels, compared with that afforded to training. This perhaps reflects what has been described as the overly academic orientation of the education system, much criticised in the 'Ruskin debate' on the relationship between education and the needs of industry,[2] combined with culturally negative attitudes towards training in the UK. Moreover, this imbalance in overall research focus is reflected in the relative degree of attention afforded to race and gender issues in critiques of the two systems. The sociology of education literature on gender and education has grown to such an extent in the UK that it now supports an entire journal of that name. However, accounts of gender issues in training are, by sharp contrast, few and far between. This chapter seeks to redress this balance by focusing on women and training issues.

THE GENDERING OF DISCOURSE AND ORGANISATION

The issue of the gendering of language was introduced in Chapter 2, where attention was drawn to the confusions and complexities of dealing with EO in a transnational context where words and meanings differ and some key terms do not exist at all in some languages. Among the civil servants of Brussels, a new language is evolving made up of borrowings from those languages that have a term for the concept the speaker wishes to convey. French words which often crop up in this respect include *acquis* and *alternance*, where no direct English equivalent exists. This section examines key terms in training policy to seek to deconstruct and reconstruct them from a more gender-aware perspective.

The first term, *skill*, is one that has already attracted considerable interest from feminist writers. Phillips and Taylor (1980) were among the first to draw attention to the relationship between the gender of those deemed to have certain occupational skills and the value attached to them (but see also Gaskell 1986; Horrell *et al.* 1990). Patterns of gender segregation are intrinsically linked with the categorisation of jobs as skilled, semi-skilled or unskilled. This in turn determines the rewards which such skills attract.

Other factors determining the social construction of skill include the power and status of the job incumbent (which are also socially constructed along gender lines). Industrial muscle has proved essential in sustaining pay differentials, even where occupations have become deskilled, as Cockburn (1983) illustrated in relation to the print industry. She shows how, even when the skill component of the tasks diminished through the introduction of new technologies and physical strength was no longer a pre-requisite, the members of the all-male union managed to continue to exclude women and sustain wage rates for a level of skill that no longer pertained. There was resistance to admitting women into the industry on the grounds that feminised occupations receive lower wages, an empirically sound observation. Mitter (1986) has also shown the strength of unions in affecting the determination of the level of skills attributed to tasks: where unions are weak or non-existent, women's work is more likely to be defined as unskilled or semi-skilled. However, unions are repeatedly shown in empirical studies to be dominated by men who set the agenda, even where the majority of members are women (Lawrence 1994).

The route through which skills are acquired is another important determinant of the extent to which they are valued. Generally, skills learned through education, training or experience are valued more than 'innate' skills (although the creative arts and sporting world are exceptions to this). And those skills which are acknowledged through certification are deemed more significant than those which are not. Hence old-style time-served apprentices, the vast majority of whom were men, enjoyed high status even where their skills might be superseded by new technologies. Of the 230,000 apprentices in Britain in the winter of 1993/4, only 20 per cent were women (LFS).[3] Women, by contrast, who learned their skills through in-house training or 'sitting-by-Nellie' – an almost untranslatable English expression indicating training where new recruits learn by watching colleagues who, in effect, act as informal trainers through example – are deemed less skilled (see Rees 1992b).

Men and women have different perceptions of the types of skills required in their jobs and of the level of skill involved, according to a study of over 600 employees by Horrell et al. (1990). Full-time male workers were more likely to think of their work as skilled than were female part-time workers. The study's authors suggest that previous research, dominated by examinations of skills in manufacturing, has led to the undermining of social and communication skills used more frequently in the service sector. In their previous work (Horrell et al. 1989) the authors found a tendency for men to occupy jobs deemed more skilled than those of women. However, full-time women workers were found to be systematically lower paid than full-time male workers, even after adjusting for any differences in the skill composition of their jobs. On the basis of their research, Horrell *et al.* (1990) conclude that 'the main cleavage in the quality or skill level of jobs is not between all male and all female jobs but between full- and part-time jobs' (p. 214). They predict that the growth of part-time work will lead to greater polarisation *among* women's skill levels, a prediction which has echoes in other studies (see Rees 1992b).

While attempts have been made by Horrell *et al.* (1990) and others to construct an index of skill to isolate its components from its gendered setting, it is clear that factors directly or indirectly related to gender associations, such as sector, unionisation, method of acquiring skill and even hours worked, impact upon the value attached to particular skills. The concept of skill is, therefore, socially constructed, and reflects power relations between the genders, which in turn are cemented in structures which systematically increase the value attached to skills in predominantly male occupations.

Second, the concept of *training* itself is highly ambiguous, so much so that Campanelli *et al.* (1994) discovered a variety of different usages in common currency. As might be expected, there is some confusion about the distinction between education and training. The general population has a narrower concept of training than that of training providers, one that is restricted to formal off-the-job training. Similarly, employers have a more restricted definition of training than employees, tending to disregard activities not initiated or funded by employers themselves (Campanelli *et al.* 1994). The net effect of this may be that certain training activities may be unreported (for example, by respondents to the LFS) and fail to be acknowledged and rewarded.

An Employment Department (ED) definition described training as 'intentional intervention to help the individual (or the organisation) to become competent, or more competent, at work.' (ED 1993: 8).[4] However, this would need to be interpreted extremely broadly if women's training workshops are to be regarded as training providers. Many such workshops targeting disadvantaged women returners may only contribute to directly employment-related competences over a long time scale. For women who are in the process of returning to work, building up sufficient confidence to enrol on standard training courses or enter employment is part of what such workshops offer. Without it, they may not return to the labour market at all, or not in a capacity which reflects their potential. Substantive skills are also taught, but trainees report that these do not provide a major motivation for enrolling (Essex *et al.* 1986). But through learning, confidence to take decisions is increased. This may mean subsequently taking an education or training course in a completely different subject, or it may mean leaving an abusive relationship, one of a series of decisions which only leads to an increase in human resources available to the labour force in the longer run (Essex *et al.* 1986; Rees 1992b). The growth in trainees' confidence may be far more significant in determining pathways of returning to the workforce than the precise nature of substantive skills learned in women's training workshops. Hence, definitions of training which are tied too closely to employment may leave out activities which operate within a much broader timescale, and where other aspects of trainees' lives are important determinants of the trajectories between training and skills available for increasing competences at work.

Third, the concepts of 'unemployment' and 'employment' are similarly gendered in their social construction (Marsh 1988). Research on women returning to training or work after a period of domestic responsibilities illustrates that they undergo a process of moving towards a state of readiness rather than experiencing a sudden shift in self-categorisation from, say, full-time carer to 'unemployed'. The ambivalence in status in relation to the labour market enshrined in some married women's ineligibility to the JSA compounds this ambiguity. Similarly, many women returners' desire for further training before entering the labour market, together with the use of informal networks to access employment opportunities, and their preference for part-time employment, further confound the description of such women as straightforwardly 'unemployed' (Hardill and Green 1990; Healy and Kraithman 1989; Martin and Roberts 1984; Sargeant 1989). The concept of unemployment and its operationalisation through the JSA system more readily suits those whose adult lives engage in the labour force without breaks for domestic commitments, and who work or seek work on a full-time basis. This applies to more men than women, and is the norm against which women's participation in the labour force is measured (Beechey 1987).

The normative use of full-time employment again relegates part-time, temporary and other forms of contractual arrangements as 'atypical', in the discourse of the EC (see, for example, Meulders *et al.* 1994). Despite the fact that such arrangements describe the basis on which millions of women in the EU engage with the labour market, they are conceived in relation to patterns which describe the nature of participation by most men. The use of the term 'atypical work' is the most glaringly obvious indication of the gendered social construction of employment. Its translation into official statistics leads systematically to the under-recording of women's contribution to the economy.

Fourth, concepts such as 'career' are also informed by a particular model of a trajectory, one followed by most men. Research on schoolgirls' option and career 'choices' illustrates that, for some, ideas about their future careers are informed by anticipation of an interrupted career which severely restricts their range of opportunities and disinclines them to invest in their own human capital (Pilcher *et al.* 1988). Even women teachers describe their 'careers' as a 'series of accidents' (Acker 1992: 3). Women in charge of their own businesses operating in more than one European country and with turnovers of over half a million pounds a year, in Muir's research, also attribute their current position to the result of a series of happenstances (Muir 1994a; 1994b; 1997).

Finally, the terms 'self-employed' and 'entrepreneur' are often used interchangeably, although the latter term is muddied in the UK with ideological concepts of the Government-encouraged, boot-strapping enterprise culture of the 1980s. The lack of clarity in definition is likely to lead to the under-counting of women who are self-employed. Women working part-time in their businesses are most likely to be unrecorded. An EC study of 17,000 'non-employed' women found that definitions of self-employment used by national governments for the compilation of statistics exclude many women who either run their own businesses or who work independently (CEC 1987a). This under-counting may lead to gaps in the provision of support services as the level of potential demand is not appreciated. Models of the entrepreneur which inform finance houses (Carter and Cannon 1988) and providers of enterprise training (Smith 1993a; 1993b) tend to be male. Ideas of 'success' in self-employment are gendered too: while both men and women may speak of independence and autonomy, for men this may mean freedom to make decisions and not be constrained, for many women it may mean a more palatable method of reconciling the time demands of home and work (Hakim 1989), or simply the only basis on which they can engage in the labour market, given its sexist and racist discriminatory practices and the constraints of domestic commitments, poverty and lack of qualifications (Phizacklea and Wolkowitz 1995).

The reconceptualisation of key terms in training and the labour market needs, of course, to move beyond pointing out their gendered social construction. The language of academic institutions gives out clear messages to both genders on who 'belongs' – from the bestowing of Bachelors' and Masters' degrees to the awarding of Fellowships. However, the male hegemony of education and training provision is also reflected in the social organisation, formal and informal curriculum and hierarchies. These combine to determine the basis on which consumers (of either gender) feel comfortable and the extent to which they feel they belong. Not only are different subjects and departments gendered to a greater or lesser extent in all these respects but institutions as a whole reflect priorities of the powerful. Decisions about what knowledge is privileged, how the timetable is constructed, and what account is taken of other aspects of gendered lives, are all crucial. At one level this can be about scheduling classes, so that fears about travelling after dark alone are accommodated or so that those with childcare responsibilities can collect their children at an appropriate time. Garland (1994), for example, reports in her study of mature-aged women students that their course choices were constrained by what was available at a time that allowed them to be back home by three thirty for the children. The gendered social construction of language around training issues is only an outward and manifest signal of the deeply gendered organisation of post-compulsory education and training

At another level, reconceptualising key terms is about shifting from being geared to one section of the population to opening doors to all. This implies imaginative strategies to manage diversity, ensuring that all consumers are made to feel they fit. Garland (1994: 115) in this respect reports how terrified mature-aged women students felt on a campus overwhelmingly made up of school-leavers:

> If that's what stress feels like I was extremely stressed, I felt ill, I had butterflies in my tummy, I couldn't eat, I lost half a stone in the first week. Anyway I stuck it out, I got worse toward the end of the first week, but then someone came up to me, another mature female student, and said 'Do you know I feel absolutely dreadful', and I realized that there were other people who felt just as bad as I did.

Similarly, some women at home with children, while aware of the need to return to education or training to improve their prospects in the labour market, express their fear of enrolling (Spencer and Taylor 1994: 17):

> I don't think I'd have the confidence nowadays. I'd feel silly. I think I'm afraid I'd make a fool of myself. It was OK when you were still at school 'cos you were used to it. But now, I just couldn't go.

Clearly, institutions which wait for such students to cross the threshold will not be as attractive as women's workshops which come to meet them halfway through outreach work.

There has been growing discontent with the male-streamism of the academic mode of production in the UK from both staff and students (see Bagihole 1993; Heward 1994; Ramazanoglu 1987).[5] This includes critiques of the extent to which inequalities in the domestic division of labour prevent women in academic life from achieving promotion in a system geared to privileging research, which increasingly has to be undertaken during hours additional to the notional forty for which staff are paid. It includes celebrations of a 'feminist space' within universities through the introduction and extension of women's studies courses (Aaron and Walby 1991; Kennedy *et al.* 1993). It also comprises articulate critiques of the academic mode of production from women students for whom educational institutions are unwelcoming places (Taking Liberties Collective 1989) and of the girl-unfriendly nature of schools (Whyte *et al.* 1985). The gendered ideology of the curriculum has also been a focus of concern (David 1983).

In training there has been far less research on these matters and far fewer critiques of the male hegemony which characterises its language, organisation and delivery. However, studies of women-only training workshops which have achieved remarkable results in equipping disadvantaged women for the labour market pick up on similar themes to those in studies of women in education. They identify the strength of their approach as lying in their 'woman centredness', (Cary 1995; Essex *et al.* 1986). This involves overcoming fears induced by lack of confidence and knowledge, addressing domestic responsibilities directly or indirectly, accommodating the facts that many women have few resources to invest in their own training or in transport to get to it, and that such women may have few contacts and networks in a changing labour market and will need tailor-made guidance and counselling.

In conclusion, the use of words, the structure and organisation of education and training organisations and the models which underpin them are highly gendered in their construction. This has important implications for what is valued and what is rewarded. If women are the majority of the low-skilled and unskilled, then this is in part a function of gendered segregation in access and take-up of training, but it is also, in part, a reflection of the patriarchal construction of what competences are regarded as skilled.

GENDER SEGREGATION IN POST-COMPULSORY EDUCATION AND TRAINING

Gender monitoring

The 'political arithmetic' tradition has made a significant contribution to our understanding of patterns of outcome from systems which seek to afford equality of access. Whether it be the influence of class on allocation of places in higher education (Halsey 1977), the impact of religion on education and employment in Northern Ireland (Cormack and Osborne 1991, 1993), or of race on performance in education (Swann 1985), such accounts provide powerful evidence of the effect of discrimination and disadvantage in social organisation.

Immediate problems faced by those seeking to conduct a political arithmetic exercise on gender and training include the ambiguity surrounding what constitutes training (discussed above) and the lack of figures presented on a gender basis (Istance and Rees 1994). A further crucial point is that there is no distinction drawn in accounts of training, for example in the LFS, between training which is potentially transformative, that is, likely to improve occupational lifechances, and that which merely facilitates people to do their current job. In other words, while some training will lead to the development of skills that enable the trainee to enhance their human capital, other forms of training merely serve the purpose of induction of a new employee, or provide instruction in health and safety at work or familiarity with new equipment, all geared to allow employees to perform their existing jobs more adequately or safely. The significance of the difference between these types of training is crucial. Failure to distinguish between them in statistical accounts can be most misleading. As women are more likely to have career breaks and return to the labour market than men, clearly a substantial proportion of the employer-sponsored training they receive may well be induction training. The length of training can be a surrogate indicator here, and it is noticeable that, while women may be the majority of the recipients of employer-sponsored training of three days or less, men are far more likely to have longer-term sponsored training (Istance and Rees 1994).

Data sources on training are problematic, although the main one, the LFS, has increased its periodicity to every three months; its sample size to allow interrogation of smaller spatial units in particular regions; and the number of questions about training. This is clearly welcome. The Youth Cohort Survey of Scotland (now also of England and Wales) provides data on young people's access to training (Payne 1994). The National Child Development Study, a longitudinal study which follows a cohort of people born in 1958, furnishes a unique insight into the gender dimension of training trajectories (Bynner and Fogelman 1993; Morphy et al. 1997). Felstead's (1996) useful secondary analysis of women's performance in New Vocational Qualifications (NVQs) (see Appendix II) illustrates a further gendered dimension to the statistical representation of women in training. As he concludes from his analysis of NVQs, and Bynner and Fogelman (1993) from their study of the National Child Development Study, women are less likely to have had their skills certificated. Hence, qualifications are 'an incomplete measure of work-related skills and a poor reflection of workers' relative abilities' (Felstead 1996: 47). The authors question the traditional association made between skills and qualifications.

The TECs set up in England and Wales and the Local Enterprise Companies (LECs) in Scotland were intended to provide both a locally sensitive response to training needs and a national network of organisations.[6] However, the opportunity for developing systematic statistical practices with built-in gender monitoring was not taken up. A review of women in post-compulsory education and training in Wales commissioned by the EOC incurred difficulties because of this (Istance and Rees 1994). All eight Welsh TECs were asked for gender breakdowns of participation in TEC-funded programmes. The replies included the following observations and remarks:

We are in the process of developing a Management Information Return that will breakdown the data sufficiently to satisfy enquiries . . . so will be unable to answer those questions at present.

It has not been possible within the timescale requested to provide more detailed information. . . .

Most of this data [on gender take-up of public training] is not readily available from our management information system . . . unfortunately our records on Enterprise and Management training are less accessible. This will not be the case for much longer. Basically, what we have tells you numbers of participants and not much else. Soon, however, our data should be similar and more robust throughout our programmes.

(Welsh TEC information officers, quoted in Istance and Rees 1994)

Within Wales there are attempts being made to systematise data following an initiative from the Welsh Office. However, for the time being, it is clear that individual TECs vary considerably in the extent to which gender monitoring data are collected, stored in an accessible form, made available externally, or indeed used internally in reviewing performance, marketing and forward planning. Gender monitoring as such clearly is not a feature of the organisation of work in the Welsh TECs, and as a consequence provision is not informed by an awareness of gender effects. Service-level agreements with TECs provide an opportunity to rectify this.

This lack of a gender dimension in published statistics is not, of course, simply a characteristic of Welsh TECs, it is an EU-wide issue. A publication issued by DGXXII as recently as 1994, giving facts and figures on higher education over a decade, misses an opportunity to illustrate gender differences and similarities (EC 1994d). Lack of systematic gender monitoring is indicative of a lack of concern about the development of women's skills, despite the pressing need indicated by the sources which are available. There are two recent developments which may indicate a change in the future, one at UK and one at EU level. Investors in People (IIP) in the UK has insisted since January 1997 that employers seeking to achieve IIP status must include gender monitoring as part of review and staff development procedures within their human resource management strategy. Second, the mainstreaming agenda in the EU will require organisations participating in EC funded programmes to have gender monitoring in place in order to fulfil reporting requirements for the administration of projects.

Women's participation in post-compulsory education and training[7]

In the UK there has been a veritable moral panic following the broadcasting of a current affairs programme on national television suggesting that girls were outperforming boys in schools (BBC TV's *Panorama*, 24 October 1994). However, a recent review of gender equality in schools in England and Wales following a series of educational reforms (Arnot *et al.* 1996; see also Salisbury 1996 on Wales) advocates caution in interpreting the statistics. Girls may in fact be 'catching up' in some fields and outperforming boys in others, but those educational successes tend not to be translated into appropriate labour market positions. Moreover, gendered analyses of women's participation and performance in vocational training, again analysed with caution, are a cause for concern, as this section seeks to demonstrate with particular reference to Wales.

The complexity of the broad trends in the position of women in education is illustrated in a recent official summary compiled by the Department for Education (1993: 1–2):

1 Girls generally achieved better results at GCSE than boys.
2 Women were more likely to participate in education at ages 16 and 17 than men. Men were more likely to be in part-time education among these age groups.
3 Women were more likely to take and pass A-levels than men. However, male candidates had a slightly better success rate.
4 Women undergraduates were more likely to study arts and humanities (including business and teacher training) and less likely to study sciences than men.
5 The unemployment rate among female graduates was much lower than among their male counterparts. The types of work which graduates entered also differed considerably between the sexes.
6 In the population as a whole men generally had a higher level of qualification than women. However, the gap was much narrower among the younger age groups.
7 There were more women teachers than men. Women were particularly numerous among primary teachers. The proportion of women was highest among younger teachers.
8 Women aged 18 or over were more likely to be participating in education than men. This was particularly true among older age groups.
9 Women were more likely to be studying on short further

education courses than men. They obtained more vocational qualifications than men but men gained more at higher levels.

This summary illustrates how important it is to explore below broad patterns of participation in order to establish the impact of gender on both subject and type and level of provision. While there has been an increase in women's level of participation, gender remains an extremely significant determinant of who gets what education and training, and consequent employment patterns.

School-based qualifications act as a filter to more advanced education and training courses. It is only relatively recently that the level of attainment in school-based qualifications has evened up between the genders, although subject differences remain starkly apparent. The most recent figures are presented in Table 5.1. This illustrates that a higher proportion of young women than young men achieve two or more A levels and that women are less likely than men to leave school with no graded results at all in England, Scotland and Wales.

However, the table also illustrates considerable variation between England, Scotland and Wales (although the gap has been closing). Wales has both extremes: high proportions of both high achievers and low achievers.

Given the collapse of the youth labour market, few Welsh school-leavers without qualifications are likely to make good this deficit through employment-related training: only 1.8 per cent of the entire female 16-year-old cohort went into a job with training in Wales in 1993 compared with 2.5 per cent of males (Istance and Rees 1994). Moreover, a study of 16 to 18-year-olds in South

Table 5.1.   School-leavers with two or more 'A' levels (three or more Highers in Scotland) and with no graded results in school qualifications([a]) in England, Scotland and Wales, 1992/93

	A levels 2+b		No graded results	
	Males	Females	Males	Females
England	20.0	21.6	11.1	8.2
Scotland	24.1	28.6	6.4	4.6
Wales	26.0	33.5	13.5	8.5

Notes: [a]Refers to GCSE, CSE, SCE, A or AS levels or Highers, but not to other vocational qualifications; [b]3 or more Highers in Scotland
Source: Calculated from Central Statistical Office (1995) *Regional Trends 30*, London: HMSO, Table 4.7

Glamorgan revealed that 12.7 per cent of males and 11.9 per cent of females in this age group 'disappear' from any contact with the careers service, schools, colleges, employers or other authorities or agencies. They are simply not to be found in education, training or employment (see Chapter 9; Istance *et al.* 1994; Rees *et al.* 1996). Such young people (the 'Youth Guarantee Group') are eligible for a place on the Government's Youth Training (YT) scheme designed to prepare them for the labour market. However, the numbers going into YT have declined, and those who do enter are more and more likely to be young men. The introduction of eligibility criteria for access to the Youth Guarantee Group, such as 'displaying appropriate attitudes', has had the effect of reducing apparent youth unemployment, and also means that we have no statistics on those who have 'disappeared'. The South Glamorgan study (which has been replicated in other parts of the UK such as the North-East of England (Wilkinson 1995) and Northern Ireland (Training and Employment Agency 1996) illustrates that more than 10 per cent of male and female 16 to 18-year-olds are likely to be increasingly difficult to count, identify, contact and coax into education, training or employment (Istance *et al.* 1994).[8]

Women make up the majority of students and trainees in further education in Wales. However, the basis on which they participate is quite different from that of men. They are much more likely to attend in the evening or through open or distance learning programmes. Only a quarter of women in FE are in part-time day courses compared with a third of the male students. Two-thirds of students on 'day-release' or 'block-release' arrangements, with close contacts with employers, are men. Women are more likely to be either on courses which do not lead to a qualification at all, or on academic courses (GCSE and A level). Men, meanwhile, are more likely to be found on vocational courses, studying for technical qualifications such as Business and Technology Education Council (BTEC) or City and Guilds (Istance and Rees 1994).

This pattern of men being more likely to be on courses directly linked to employment is reflected in the patterns of segregation shown in the growing non-university higher education sector. Men are the majority of students on sandwich or release courses. There is a more or less even gender distribution in some subjects. However, others, such as mathematics and computing, architecture and building, and engineering and technology, remain clearly male preserves, while education and medically-related courses are numerically dominated by women.

Access courses have mushroomed in recent years in Wales, as in the rest of the UK: there was a ten-fold expansion in numbers between 1988/9 and 1993/4. Approximately three-quarters of access students in Wales progress to higher education. Women constitute some 58 per cent of access students in Wales, some of whom are from the missing generation of women undergraduates from the 1950s and 1960s. The range of courses to which access students progress remains largely limited to arts and humanities: in particular, very few study science. This is despite the fact that many institutions run a 'preliminary' year for students on science and engineering courses: these do not exist in the arts and social sciences.

At undergraduate level, women students in Wales now slightly outnumber men, although there are more male than female graduates: the catch-up in enrolment has been quite recent. However, once again there are significant patterns of gender segregation within degree courses. Women have increased in numbers on professional courses such as business and administration, law and accountancy, and have sustained a high representation in arts, social sciences, education and medically-related fields. However, they remain very thin on the ground in science, technology and engineering. Women in the University of Wales are under-represented in science, not simply in relation to men, but compared with women in other parts of the UK[9] (Istance and Rees 1994). It is clear, then, that women are participating more in academic courses than they were, and in some fields achieve more qualifications than men, albeit in a limited range of subjects. However, in non-degree-level vocational courses, the gap between men and women appears to be widening.

The Confederation of British Industry (CBI) has been a prime mover in the drive for credentialism in the UK, the recognition of skills through awarding certificates (CBI 1989). It noted in 1989 that South Korea was aiming that 80 per cent of its young people should reach university entrance standard by the end of the century, and that France had set a target of 75 per cent. Equivalent actual figures for the UK at the time were 30 per cent reaching university entrance standard and 15 per cent entering higher education. The Trades Union Congress has also voiced support for the development of skills (TUC 1989). The Government introduced National Targets for Education and Training (NTETs) to combine academic and vocational qualifications and to express them in terms of NVQ equivalents.[10] There are four such levels, broadly equivalent to academic levels (see Appendix II). These qualifications have replaced the rather complex set of qualifications previously offered by the range of accreditation bodies. The qualification indicates that an individual is able to perform a job in a particular occupation to a specified skill level. So far, there are 500 NVQs in 150 occupations. However, employer awareness of them remains low, especially among small and medium-size enterprises (SMEs).

Targets have been set at national, regional and TEC/LEC area level (DfEE/Scottish Office/Welsh Office 1995). A distinction is made between Foundation Targets (FTs) for young people and Lifetime Targets (LTs) for adults. Of all the regions of England and countries of the UK relating to FT Level Target 1 qualifications attained by 19–21-year-olds (FT1 is at least NVQ level 2 or equivalent), the Welsh figures are the lowest. Compared with the UK average on FT1 of 61 per cent, 58 per cent attained this level in Wales (NACETT 1994, Annex 1, Table 1). However, in contrast to the other parts of the UK, the female rate is higher than that of males in Wales (Istance and Rees 1996).

The Youth Cohort Study for England and Wales shows that young women are more likely to gain Royal Society of Arts (RSA) qualifications in clerical and related subjects (NVQ level 1 equivalent) while young men gain BTEC or City and Guilds in craft and related subjects (mostly NVQ level 2) (Payne 1994). Comments from the report of the National Advisory Council for Education and Training Targets (NACETT) for the UK as a whole identified the differential attainment of academic and vocational qualifications as crucial in accounting for the common pattern of gender differences, based in this case on England:

> In England, girls continue to out perform boys at GCSE (by about seven percentage points). But overall, 4% fewer girls than boys are reaching the Foundation Target 1 level. This implies that the proportion of girls achieving level 2 vocational qualifications is about two-thirds that of boys. The Council believes that further research on girls' take-up of vocational qualifications is needed so that those responsible for the development of GNVQs and NVQs can take early action to address this apparent imbalance.
>
> (NACETT 1994: 17)

Wales is behind the other UK countries and all the English regions in the proportion of 21-year-olds achieving FT3 (that is, at least NVQ level 3 or equivalent) (31 per cent as against a UK average of 37 per cent (NACETT 1994, Annex 1, Table 7). Gender breakdowns are not available in the regional analysis, but the situation in England overall gives cause for concern as regards women's access to and take-up of vocational training at this level too:

> There is a significant difference – of ten percentage points – between the overall achievement levels of young men and women. Comparison of their respective GCE A level achievements suggests that, compared with males, comparatively few females are pursuing and succeeding in level 3 vocational qualifications. Also, there is a wider gap between males and females at level 3 than at level 2. This suggests that fewer females who could benefit, are successfully undertaking level 3 courses. It is clear that – as part of the drive to strengthen vocational routes – more should be done to make suitable vocational qualifications available to, and attractive to, young women so as to encourage them to continue their education and training beyond level 2.
>
> (NACETT 1994: 25)

One of the major problems for women in the drive for credentialism is that it means funding has been withdrawn from non-credited courses in further and continuing education and training (that is, courses not leading to a qualification). This may well deter women returners who lack the confidence to move straight into credited courses for fear of failing. At the very stage when the EC is encouraging the creation of more ports of entry into vocational education and training systems and improving routes of progression between systems (EC 1996b), the first rung on the ladder of returning to learn has in effect been removed in the UK. On the other hand, the extension of opportunities for the Accreditation of Prior Learning (APL) is clearly likely to benefit women whose skills acquired through voluntary sector activities are not formally recognised. It will be necessary to be vigilant to ensure that the gendered construction of skill does not result in the gendering of accreditation: this would result in the discounting or undervaluing of 'women's' skills as opposed to 'men's'. Hence, women with accredited skills in female dominated areas may find they become ghettoised within those fields and encounter difficulties in transferring to other training opportunities. While it is too early to judge the overall effect of this policy of credentialism on women, it is clear that there are already some real and potential weaknesses.

Just under 10 per cent of the population of working age in Britain received job-related training in the four weeks prior to one of the data collection periods in the LFS in 1992, but, again, the figure for Wales was only 8.6 per cent (DE 1993: Table B21). The LFS does not ask about the types or length of training received, which can be highly significant. The reports of an increase in job-related training for women in the LFS would need further analysis to establish the extent to which it is truly transformative. For example, in Spring 1994 the LFS shows that unemployed women in Britain were more likely than unemployed men to have received job-related training in the last four weeks (9 per cent compared with 6 per cent). However, women were more likely to have paid their fees themselves or had them paid by relatives (37 per cent compared with 32 per cent), and less likely to have had their fees paid by the Government or a local authority (41 per cent compared with 48 per cent).

An important aspect to the gendering of employer-sponsored training is the extent to which it is informed by expectations of mobility within the company. In a study of a hundred employees (fifty/fifty men and women) working for six employers in South Wales, access to training was closely linked to the status of the employee (Rees *et al.* 1991). Hence, managers, supervisors and employees in the craft technician category were far more likely to have received training than those in the (largely female) sectors of clerical/secretarial and production operative grades. As a result, a quarter of the female respondents had received no training at all in recent years, compared with only a handful of the men. This is unsurprising and illustrates how segregation in training underpins and reinforces segregation in employment and vice versa. However, the significant point for us here, and one that is crucial in interpreting data on access to and participation in training, is that the *type* of training received by men and women in the same occupational group varied substantially. In the managers/supervisors group, women's training was overwhelmingly up-dating or retraining, while that of men was more likely to be directed towards the acquisition of qualifications and career development (Rees *et al.* 1991, 1992). In other words, training for men increased their occupational lifechances, while that for women merely enabled them to carry out their current jobs. This illustrates the need to explore the nature of training received by men and women in addition to issues around access and participation.

In conclusion, while women are participating more in post-compulsory education and succeeding in academic courses such as GCSEs, A levels, diplomas and degrees, they remain clustered in female dominated subject areas. And as yet they are not benefiting to the same extent from vocational education and training, in particular from courses which have received employer sponsorship or are clearly linked to the labour market. As a consequence, their opportunities to use their skills and have them recognised are limited. The proportion of women in top jobs in all sectors is woefully low, even in those professions such as law, where operating the 'qualifications lever' (Crompton and Sanderson 1990b) has secured them access. Moreover, this section illustrates that there are clear locational variations in men and women's academic and voca-tional educational achievements. Wales stands out as the part of Britain where women are least likely to have vocational qualifica-tions, and where there are pitifully few women in top jobs (Rees and Fielder 1992).

CONCLUSION

This chapter has explored the gendered dimension of post-compulsory education and training in the UK ,with special reference to Wales. It has highlighted some of the effects of a specific set of economic circumstances combined with a Government policy of credentialism and marketisation of training. It has shown that the language and organisation of training are geared more towards men than women, and to full-time workers rather than to part-time employees or to women embarking on the return to learning, employment or self-employment. Gender moni-toring systems are non-existent, inadequate, unused or under-utilised in performance measurement or forward planning (although there are some limited signs of improvement as a result of initiatives from NACETT, IIP, DfEE, Scottish Office and Welsh Office). Recent changes appear on current evidence to be not thought through in terms of their gender implications, and in cases may well have detrimental effects upon women.

The underlying point of the chapter is that policies and provi-sions that are thought to be gender-neutral can have highly gendered effects. This underlines the need for a mainstreaming approach which would address not simply the differences between men and women, but also the differences among men, and the differences among women. Policies geared towards upskilling the workforce need to take on board the differences and similarities that exist among its members in order to be effective. Otherwise, the net effect of post-compulsory education and training is to solidify gender segregation in the labour market. The equal access approach, even when tempered with some positive action initiatives, does not lead to equal outcome: on the contrary, it reinforces divisions and cements gendered trajectories.

Chapter 6

Skill shortages, women, and training for the new information technologies

At the European Commission conference on Lifelong Learning for the Information Society held in Genoa, Italy in March 1996 and attended by over 500 delegates, some unfortunate technical difficulties were experienced. The conference was held to mark the European Year of Lifelong Learning and to launch a report offering the first reflections of the EC's high-level group of experts, *Building the European Information Society for Us All* (High Level Group of Experts 1996). The report sets out a vision for the future on information and communication technologies in the widest terms. The chair of the high-level expert group, Professor Luc Soete from the University of Limburg, was invited to give a presentation on growth, competitiveness and employment in the information society at the conference, in what was clearly intended to be the first show-piece dissemination of the group's views. The session was chaired by Franco Malerba, an Italian astronaut who is now a Member of the European Parliament. However, even their combined expertise, alas, proved insufficient to prepare them or the expert audience for the failure of technology during the presentation.

Soon after Professor Soete began his address from the rostrum, flanked by large, cinema-style screens on either side for the benefit of those sitting at the back of the huge auditorium, the voice of the Italian interpreter could be heard, loud and clear, emanating from the microphone on the table in front of Mr Malerba. Indeed, the disembodied but much magnified voice was somewhat louder than that of the speaker. Mr Malerba, shielding his eyes from the glare of the spotlights, looked in vain in the direction of the audience for a technician. None materialised. Some time elapsed, during which Professor Soete attempted to compete with the incorporeal voice from the microphone. Eventually, Torben Andersen from the

Odense Steel Shipyard, who was programmed to be the second speaker in the session, could bear it no longer. He walked round the table and ripped all the wires from the back of the microphone in an admittedly Luddite but nevertheless effective gesture. The voice was silenced. The tension evaporated. The audience settled back to concentrate on Professor Soete's delivery.

However, not long after this, a technician did appear. He was clearly put out at the unorthodox approach to the technical problem exercised by Mr Andersen. After some remonstration, he reconnected the wires to the microphone. Members of the audience held their collective breath. The microphone maintained its silence. The technician left. The Professor's words could still be clearly heard and the audience's attention reverted to them wholeheartedly. But to everyone's horror, minutes later, the voice of the Italian interpreter began once again to reverberate from the renegade microphone. Professor Soete bravely continued, with higher volume, his visible discomfiture magnified on the big screens on either side of the conference hall. Mr Malerba was clearly exasperated. The Danish shipping magnate boldly repeated his low-tech but effective disconnection tactic. The technician reappeared, repeated his remonstration only with rather more fervour, reconnected the wires and disappeared again. This time the voice mercifully remained confined, as intended, to the ears of those wearing headphones tuned into the Italian channel. However, by this time, Professor Soete had finished his address. The chair thanked him, and apologised for the 'technical difficulties' that had marred his presentation.

The purpose of introducing this chapter with a description of this excruciating and highly ironic episode is to point up some of the many paradoxes it encapsulates. On the one hand, new technologies allow the spread of information to a wider audience, in this case with full sound and vision and simultaneous translation into all the languages of the European Union. The ownership of knowledge of how to store, access, retrieve and utilise information more generally in the information society is spreading from the few to the many. The level of skills required to use the new technologies is lower than that which was needed, say, in the transition from a non-literate to a literate society. And yet, the capacity for mechanical malfunction and human error increases exponentially. The frustration and stress resulting from being unable to control technology is one of the most intransigent and frustrating yet neglected features of the information society.

Moreover, control over technology is highly gendered. Education, training and employment, both in technological fields but also in the growing numbers of areas which now incorporate the use of technologies, are expanding considerably. But it is largely men who are taking up and benefiting from these opportunities. Indeed, Spender argues that men are not only writing the rules of the road for the information highway, they are also subjecting women to new forms of virtual reality sexual harassment and even data rape (Spender 1995). It is women in particular who are experiencing the helplessness and frustration of being technically dependent upon others exemplified by that so cruelly faced by those under the spotlight in Genoa.

The EC White Paper *Teaching and Learning: Towards the Learning Society* (EC 1996b) emphasises that it is important for individuals to become proficient and confident in learning to use new technologies in order to access the information society. It is not simply in working life that such proficiencies bestow advantages. For individuals as consumers, campaigners and participants in public life more generally, access to and proficiency in electronic communication in particular is becoming increasingly important. The issue of access to opportunities to develop these skills is therefore clearly crucial. Gaps will widen between those who can and those who cannot participate in the information society.

The fact that new information technologies (NITS) are gendered is almost completely ignored in the White Paper on Teaching and Learning (EC 1996b, see chapter 9), despite their significance for women's occupational lifechances and participation in public life. The new technology industries are already characterised by rigid patterns of gender segregation. As more and more workers are expected to be proficient in accessing and using information through technological means, labour market opportunities for women who do not have these skills will shrink. In order to achieve lifelong learning for an information society, the issue of the gendering of technologies needs to be addressed seriously.

This is a particularly important issue, given that skill shortages are already being identified as an impediment to the exploitation of NITs, and therefore to the international competitiveness of the EU and its constituent Member States. Demographic changes imply a growing dependence upon women as a source of labour in the future, but women are less likely than men to be qualified in subjects relevant to the NITs, or to be employed in those areas where there are already chronic skill shortages. Indeed, research evidence from many Member States reports an increasing bifurcation of skill level between men and women as a result of the introduction and development of new technologies. This is clearly a cause for concern. What are the barriers to women's recruitment to training and employment in NITs? What policies could be introduced or supported to facilitate the entry of women to NITs generally and those areas of skill shortages specifically? What is being done at the European level to encourage training providers, employers and others to adapt their policies and practices to make NITs more accessible to women?

Patterns of gendering in the new technologies cannot be isolated from more general structures, mechanisms and processes which lead to a workforce which is highly segregated by gender (see Chapter 2). However, the 'masculinisation' of technology adds a complex and difficult layer (Cockburn 1983, 1985, 1986; Wajcman 1991). This chapter examines key blockages in education, training and work organisation which reinforce gender divisions in NITs. It then focuses on three areas of skill shortage identified by Virgo (1991): technicians, 'hybrids' or business analysts, and business managers. It concludes with some observations about the past and potential role of the EU in addressing this issue.

The influence of NITs is increasingly all-pervasive, both at work and at home. Computer-related jobs are the fastest-growing sector of the economy. Moreover, such skills are now required even in sectors and occupations not historically associated with their use. Front-of-house hotel receptionists, car mechanics, even academics now rely on new technologies to record, store and access information. The service sector, as well as manufacturing and construction, relies on NITs in order to be more efficient, to improve the quality and design of products and services and to increase access to information. There is growing emphasis on customer care, quality assurance and flexible 'just-in-time' production systems rather than on Tayloristic mass production. The consequence of these changes is a radical shift in patterns of work organisation for many employers. Many of the low-skilled jobs are disappearing, for example in telecommunications, construction and manufacturing (Senker and Senker 1994a, 1994b, 1994c). This is leading to job losses in low paid, low skilled, repetitive jobs which are disproportionately undertaken by women.

The NITs, combined with other changes in the labour market,

create opportunities for re-shaping patterns of work organisation and for allowing employees more scope for using their potential in their jobs. This necessarily implies a much more important role for training, in particular continuing training. The evolution of job content means that initial training will no longer suffice as a preparation for a working life. Continuing training will need to become a reality and expectation for workers and employers. Given that, between now and the end of the century, increased reliance will be put upon women already of working age, and given that they are less likely to have substantive training than men, there are considerable adaptations to be made to training provision to render it suitable for their needs. Such adaptation will be necessary in the longer term to render training suitable for older people more generally.

To what extent are NITs and other challenges opening up opportunities? To what extent are existing patterns of 'job gendering' simply overlaying the new technologies, limiting the use made of them, and stifling the potential they can offer? Many domestic users of home PCs use them only for computer games or as a typewriter that corrects spelling mistakes. So, too, but with much more serious consequences, business managers may be ignorant of the scope of NITs, despite having invested heavily in hardware. Such ignorance can lead to deskilling rather than upskilling, with women in particular finding their jobs less rewarding instead of more challenging. Such managerial short-sightedness exacerbates existing skill shortages.

In this chapter, developments in the gendering of technology in school, in education and training, and in jobs using computing skills, are reviewed. Computing is clearly not the only means of accessing the information society, but it is a key mechanism and more readily identifiable in published statistics. The key questions I wish to address are as follows:

- Why is it that girls' experiences at home and in school appear to put them off computing and give them the clear idea that this is 'male territory'?
- Why is it that, in some Member States, the number of women university students in computing has been falling whereas opportunities for employment in computing itself and for those with computing skills has been expanding?
- How will the gendering of technology impede efforts to fill skill shortages in new technologies? More specifically, how will women who take career breaks re-enter the labour market in an

information society when the gap between their outdated skills and those of employees who are continually retraining grows ever wider?

There are three categories of explanation; those which explore women's relative lack of access to NITs broadly (except at the lowest levels); those which examine barriers to women's access to those specific jobs identified as skill shortages in NITs; and those which are rooted in the masculinisation of technologies – the 'social shaping' of technologies (Wajcman 1991; Webster 1996).[1] These explanations cut across one another and all feature in the following sections on the gendering of technology in education, training and employment. The gendering of technology has serious implications, both for women's opportunities and for chronic skill shortages in the EU.

THE GENDERING OF TECHNOLOGY IN SCHOOLS

By an early age, children can identify which jobs are 'appropriate' for men and women in the labour market and which roles in the home; this knowledge informs their own sense of identity and worth, it influences decisions they make about what subjects to take at school, their responses to further education and training opportunities, and their expectations of their role in the family (Holland 1988). In short, gender influences the investment that young people make in their own human capital, the subject of the qualifications they will seek to acquire, and the extent to which they will choose a job or career expected to sustain themselves, and perhaps a family, for life. Girls' expectations of their futures as mothers affect their attitudes to training and employment (see Rees 1992b: chapter 3).

Why girls show a particular aversion to computing has been the subject of considerable debate. Attitudes towards computing are clearly formed early on, largely under the twin influences of home and school. At home, research evidence suggests that parents are much more likely to buy home computers for their sons than for their daughters (Newton 1991). Wajcman (1991: 54) claims that boys are identified as the clear target by designers of computer games:

Games are the primary attraction for children. Given that it is men (often computer hackers) who design video games and software, it is hardly surprising that their designs typically appeal to male fantasies. Many of the most popular games today are simply programme versions of traditionally male non-computer games, involving shooting, blowing up, speeding or zapping in some way or another. They often have militaristic titles such as 'Destroy all Subs' and 'Space Wars' highlighting their themes of adventure and violence. No wonder then that these games often frustrate or bore the non-macho players exposed to them. As a result macho males often have a positive first experience with the computer; other males and most females have a negative initial experience.

Wajcman argues that video games have taken over from pinball machines in amusement arcades which have always been regarded as male territory, with girls looking on. New technologies are therefore clearly confirmed as male territory in adolescence.

This view is reinforced at school. Some writers have noted that the introduction of computers in schools was immediately followed by their colonisation as male territory. Despite the fact that computers can trace their ancestry through languages, communication and logic (arguably identifiable as 'female' areas) as well as science and mathematics (more overtly 'male' subjects), schools tend to locate computers in mathematics departments, although they could arguably, given their genesis, just as logically be placed in language departments (Pelgrum and Plomp 1991). Computing studies tend to be taught by male maths teachers, even though it is now widely recognised that a predilection for maths is not an essential prerequisite to computing (TFHR 1991).

Computer use in schools was found to be male-dominated throughout the education systems of nineteen countries included in one highly detailed study (Pelgrum and Plomp 1991). In all but the French-speaking countries, less than 50 per cent of the schools had a special policy concerning computing and gender issues. Where there was such a policy, it tended to be directed to training female teachers in computing education, in other words, fostering female role models. The study showed that female teachers responsible for computing in schools were rarer than female Principals in charge of schools.

For older children, evidence from all the (then twelve) Member States (see Rees 1990) illustrated that gender plays a significant role in determining what subjects girls and boys take at school: it is the single most important determinant of option choice. Despite a plethora of special initiatives designed to encourage girls into, for example, science and computing, sex stereotyping in subject choice remains highly potent. As a recent evaluation of special projects in the European Community reported:

> Students' attitudes to technology were found to be very much along traditional lines: boys prefer technical tasks; girls lack confidence; girls are reluctant to use computers; boys display dominant behaviour in the computer room.
>
> (TFHR 1990: 4)

Schools that have instituted girl-only computer clubs report some success in overcoming the effects of the dominance of computer lessons by boys. It is, of course, also well known that girls attending single-sex schools are less likely to manifest gender-stereotyped subject preferences than those in co-educational schools (Deem 1984). There is evidence, too, that boys and girls have different learning styles towards computing: girls seek to 'understand' computers while boys want to 'master' them (Davidson and Cooper 1987; Dick and Faulstich-Wieland 1988). However, it is not clear to what extent this finding is addressed in the pedagogy of schools.

In the UK, Durndell and Thomson (1997) report that, over a ten-year period, the gender gap in proficiency in computing has widened among new entrants to a British university. One of the reasons for young women being put off computers was reported as the 'silly and immature' violent computer games, referred to above. In Germany, as elsewhere, fewer girls than boys take computing and mathematics at school and female participation diminishes rapidly with age, hence fewer girls have the necessary qualifications to be taken on as apprentices (Schiersmann 1988). Similarly, throughout the EU, relatively few girls leave with appropriate qualifications to progress to higher education in computing studies.

WOMEN AND COMPUTING IN POST-COMPULSORY EDUCATION AND TRAINING

Women comprise less than half the undergraduate population (49 per cent in 1991/2, Eurostat 1995a: 111) and considerably less than half the post-graduate population in the EU. Women in higher education are more likely than men to be following short courses (Eurostat 1992: 61). As women are unlikely to possess qualifications in appropriate subjects to enrol on degree courses leading to high-level IT work, they have always been in the minority of students on computing studies degrees at university in the EU.

However, curiously enough, while the proportion of women enrolling in computer studies degree courses is increasing in some of the southern countries, notably Spain and Portugal, there is a decline in some of the more northern Member States such as Germany, Italy, Belgium and the UK. It is of particular concern that the proportion of female computing studies students in the UK dropped from about 25 per cent in the 1970s to 12 or 13 per cent in the 1980s (Rubery *et al.* 1992: Table 2.b.4.). This is at the very time when labour market opportunities in this field have been increasing so significantly. A further cause for concern is that women in the new German Länder are especially poorly represented in courses in computer science (Rubery and Fagan 1993). Moreover, it is not simply in computing studies that women are in the minority: other related disciplines show a similar picture:

> whatever progress has been made towards achieving greater equality between the sexes in general education, it remains over-whelmingly the case that women are under-represented at all levels (and especially in post-compulsory education) in those disciplines which are most closely associated with new ITs – computing, mathematics, physics and engineering.
>
> (OECD 1986, quoted in Rees 1990: 15)

In those courses particularly associated with the NITs, women range from just over a third of all students in natural sciences, and under a third in mathematics and computing, to only 9 per cent in engineering (see Table 6.1).

Engineering is an area where there are skill shortages in the EU. In the mid-1980s, the proportion of women in higher education among those studying engineering varied from very low proportions in Luxembourg (2.7 per cent) and the UK (4.1 per cent) to much higher proportions in Portugal (17 per cent) and France (16.1 per cent) (Eurostat 1992: 61, 1984 figures). In 1991/2, the proportion of women students in higher education in the EU who were studying engineering was 6 per cent, compared with 29 per cent of men, while the figure for natural sciences and mathematics was 7 per cent compared with 13 per cent of men (Eurostat 1995a: 116) (EU12 except Portugal and Luxembourg).

One of the main difficulties here is that restricted ports of entry to higher education in computing, engineering and the sciences, and

Table 6.1.   Students in IT-related degree and postgraduate degree
courses in the EU: percentage women 1985/86

	Natural sciences	Mathematics and Computer science	Engineering
Belgium	39.6 (combined)		11.9
Denmark	30.4	22.9	12.0
Federal Republic of Germany	30.9	23.6	6.5
Greece	37.0	36.0	19.7
Spain	45.5	37.5	10.7
France	32.5	17.0	16.1
Italy	53.4	43.3	54.7
Netherlands	23.0	14.4	8.4
Portugal	63.8	54.0	22.0
UK	32.1 (combined)		8.7
Europe 12	36.6	30.0	9.0

Notes: No figures are available for Ireland and Luxembourg. These headings
refer to ISCED Fields 42, 46 and 54. Figures include full and part-time students
Source: Calculated from Tables 4 and 5, Eurostat (1988) 'Rapid Reports:
Population and social conditions (occasional), 1988: 1', *Full Time Education in
the European Community in 1985/6* Luxembourg: Eurostat

the stipulation of entry qualifications in related subjects, mean that
it is difficult for women to enter such courses later in life. It is much
easier and more common to enter higher education as a mature
student in the arts and social sciences, despite the fact that some
science departments now offer foundation years. Hence these low
figures of women science and engineering students are unlikely to
be much improved through the growing opportunities for second-
chance education.

Are there opportunities in training systems for women to 'catch
up' on computing skills after entering employment? Unfortunately,
the LFS shows us that the employees most likely to be given
employer sponsorship for medium to long-term training are people
who are already technically qualified or who hold managerial positions. Women are much less likely than men to be in either group.
By contrast, they are more likely to be sent on short induction or
health and safety courses, or offered instruction in firm-specific
equipment or software courses (see Chapter 5). In short, VET
systems need a radical rethink in order to open up routes for
women, and older women in particular, to fill skill shortages in
NITs. This creation of new progression routes and ladders
connecting education, training and employment is a theme in the

White Paper, *Teaching and Learning: Towards a Learning Society* (EC 1996b), discussed in Chapter 9.

Despite the overall disappointing scores of women in the political arithmetic of computing studies and employment within the Member States, considerable success has been achieved by women-only workshops in training women in technological subjects, including computing, throughout the EU. Here, women's fears of computing, and of technology more generally, are overcome through demystification. Pedagogically appropriate techniques are combined with confidence-building and de-stereotyping. Women's domestic commitments are taken into account in the design and delivery of the courses. This might mean adopting hours that fit in with childcare requirements, or the innovative use of distance learning.

The EC has supported many of these initiatives directly through the ESF and the action programmes, through the activities of WITEC (Women into Technology, part of the COMETT programme), through NOW (New Opportunities for Women) and through IRIS, the European network of women's training projects, all of which are described elsewhere in this book. However, overall, women constitute less than half the recipients of training opportunities from the ESF (Chapter 8), and the net effect of the EC's Community Action Programmes on training has been to widen the skill gap between men and women (Chapter 7). Women are a relatively small proportion of those who have benefited from technologically advanced training in the programmes.

It is noticeable that many of those workshops which have secured EC funding and which enjoy a high success rate in integrating women into more advanced technological courses or directly into employment, tend to be outside mainstream education and training provision. They frequently rely upon precarious funding from a range of partners that has to be secured on a year-by-year basis. They report a shortage of women trainers in computing and there is no career structure for such women within this sector. It is difficult to acquire up-to-date, expensive equipment. Providing on-site childcare is very costly. The next stage must surely be to provide more established futures for these initiatives and to graft what has been learnt from them onto the pedagogy, curriculum and organisation of mainstream provision.

Having women trainers and role models appears to be effective. A curriculum that is problem-based rather than more abstract engages women more. Interactive learning programmes which allow women to work at their own pace inspire confidence. Work placements give confidence to women trainees, and give employers experience of women doing technological work. Provision needs to be built around the fact that the return to work after a period of child-rearing or unemployment can be a long-drawn-out process. It involves juggling home and work responsibilities and gaining sufficient confidence to be pro-active in making informed decisions. Guidance and counselling is important to developing appropriate trajectories based on full information. The facts that relatively few women can afford fees, or private transport, that they bear the major commitment for the care of children and the elderly and other domestic responsibilities, and that some areas are felt by women not to be safe especially at night, all need to be taken into account. New routes of progression need to be opened up between different levels of education, training and employment to accommodate the late starts and fragmented 'careers' of women. Even those women who already have high-level qualifications lose confidence while out of the workplace and face difficulties in returning to work.

WOMEN AND EMPLOYMENT IN THE NITs

It might be argued that the new jobs evolving as a result of the NITs should provide opportunities to break down the rigidities of segregation. There is no history of association of one or other gender with a specific job for school-leavers, employees and employers to challenge. Moreover, there is less need for brawn and more for brain, and jobs associated with NITs have a cleaner image compared with some of the older male-dominated industries, such as heavy manufacturing, steel and coal. Nevertheless, new systems of segregation are already emerging within the NITs, and gender remains a potent organising principle which survives the shifts and changes that organisations are experiencing as a result of their introduction. New patterns of gender segregation are emerging within the new technologies: indeed IT is more gendered now than it used to be. Whereas computing attracted large numbers of women in the 1960s, particularly as computer programmers, it has since become 'defeminised' in many Member States.

Women comprised less than 30 per cent of computer professionals in the EU in 1990, and in most countries constituted less than 20 per cent (Rubery and Fagan 1993: 70). However, while the proportion is increasing in some Member States, especially France and Spain, it is actually decreasing in others such as Germany, Italy, Belgium and the UK, corresponding to the fall referred to earlier in the number of women students (Rubery and Fagan 1993). Table 6.2, reproduced from Rubery and Fagan's analysis of occupational segregation, uses a number of sources to calculate the share of women among computer professionals and related occupations by Member State. The higher proportion of women in some of the southern Member States can be clearly seen, reflecting the figures for female participation in higher education in these fields.

Wajcman (1991: 158) reminds us that the very first computer programmers were women and that, between 1940 and 1950, many women were engaged in programming, coding or working as machine operators:[2]

> It was because programming was initially viewed as tedious clerical work of low status that it was assigned to women. As the complex skills and valuing of programming were increasingly recognized, it came to be considered creative, intellectual and demanding 'men's work'. Thus, depending upon circumstances, different cognitive styles may be characterized as 'masculine' or 'feminine' according to the power and status that attaches.

Where trade unions are weak or non-existent, women's work is more likely to be defined as unskilled or semi-skilled (Mitter 1986). But unions, of course, are largely male-dominated institutions (even where the majority of members are women); they can be instrumental in defending the status of skilled work remaining attached to men's jobs that have actually become deskilled (see Cockburn 1983, 1985).

Of course, there is considerable vertical, as well as horizontal, segregation by gender within the labour market, and the computing field is no exception. Wellington (1989) describes six categories of 'IT task' (there are other formulations) which are set out in Table 6.3. Women predominate in the bottom two categories. There are few routes of progression from those two bottom tiers to the top ones. Ports of entry to the more highly skilled jobs require different sets of qualifications and work histories from the bottom tiers: in effect, a woman would need to leave the organisation, acquire the

Table 6.2. Share of women among computer professionals and related occupations

Member state	Statisticians, mathematicians, systems analysts and related[a] Eurostat 1990, ISCO 08	Computer professionals			
		All	analysts	analyst/ programmers	programmers
Belgium	17	13 (1981)			
Denmark	28	29 (1991)			
Germany	22	21 (1989)			
Greece	31		11 (1980)	19 (1980)	
Spain	26		25[a] (1992)		45[a] (1992)
France	22	22 (1990)			
Ireland	27	28 (1986)			
Luxembourg	12				
Netherlands	13		8 (1991)		13 (1991)
Portugal	28				
UK	20	20 (1989)	29 (1992)		23 (1992)

Note: [a] public sector only
Source: Rubery, J. and Fagan, C. (1993) Occupational Segregation of Women and Men in the European Community Brussels: DGV, Commission of the European Communities, p. 71

appropriate qualifications and seek to re-enter in order to move up the ladder.

Women are reported as having a high share of lower-level programming jobs, for which a decline in demand is anticipated (Rubery and Fagan 1993). However, in the Netherlands, while only 9 per cent of systems analysts and 13 per cent of computer programmers are women (Tijdens 1991), there are noticeable trends of women moving into professional positions and decreasing their share of the operator occupations:

> women are indeed making inroads into the high-status and fast-expanding computer professions, whereas their share among the low-status, declining operator occupations has slightly diminished.
>
> (Plantenga and Tijdens 1995: 25)

Exclusionary mechanisms operate both within the IT industry (Tierney 1995; Woodfield 1994), and elsewhere in organisations increasingly affected by the introduction and development of NITs (Eriksson *et al.* 1991). There are specific difficulties facing women seeking entry to skill shortages in NITs because of the association of technical competence with the male gender (Cockburn and Ormrod 1993: 151), and the masculinity of the cultures surrounding NITs (Cringely 1992). Moreover, Webster (1996: 34) has pointed up the social shaping of technology in both the process of technological development (through horizontal and vertical gender segregation in the IT industry) and the products, which are designed for a gender segregated workforce.

Lack of appropriate qualifications has been held to explain in part why women do not secure access to certain professional jobs, particularly those in the NITs. As professions seek to upgrade them-

Table 6.3.   Categories of IT task

Category	IT task
1	systems analysts, engineers, software engineers, designers etc.
2	programmers
3	management administration and planning
4	operators
5	secretarial, WP, stock control, clerical and office VDU users etc.
6	data preparation, data entry etc.

Source: Wellington (1989:156)

selves, they restrict entry and insist upon recognised qualifications before granting membership of a professional institution, without which it is difficult to practise. Insistence on more formal qualifications can be helpful to women in theory: the criteria are clear, and if satisfied, access to the profession is difficult to deny. This process is known as credentialism. There has certainly been an increase in women's access to the professions with the growth of credentialism. However, Crompton and Sanderson (1990a) in their studies in France and the UK have shown that, while women may secure access to male dominated professions by acquiring the necessary qualifications, patterns of segregation merely emerge *within* them. So, for example, in medicine, women are confined to the low-prestige specialisms, and have little prospect of advancing further up the hierarchy. This is paralleled in IT employment where women in one South Wales study no sooner gained access to a tier of employment where they acted as 'troubleshooters' for a company's IT system than the post was downgraded, the pay reduced and opportunities for further promotion removed (Fielder and Rees 1991).

Part of the reason for women's lack of progress in the IT industry is that the profession will make little concession to domestic responsibilities. This is similar to Massey's (1993) findings in a study of scientists where the cultural expectation in terms of time commitment meant that the male scientists not only failed to make a full contribution to domestic responsibilities but relied upon their wives to look after their needs as well. While women researchers in science and technology in France, Denmark, Greece, Portugal, Spain and the new German Länder are described as seeking to establish their careers before starting families (Collin 1992), in the Netherlands they are reported as remaining single (Stolte-Heiskanen *et al.* 1991). Cringely's (1992) account of life in the software company Microsoft makes it clear that the long hours which characterise the computing industry had led to a culture of 'singledom', not only for women but for men as well.

Studies of women who do succeed in male-dominated fields – and there are now a number of collections of interviews with such 'tall poppies', as they are known in Australia (Mitchell 1984; Watson 1989) – reveal that many tend to be child-free and have uninterrupted careers. In other words, their life and work career patterns are like those of men: they take no career breaks for childbearing and rearing, they are able to move for a promotion, and they can accommodate the needs of a 'greedy' institution (Kanter

1976) which demands they work long hours and prioritise the needs of the job over any personal commitments. While such women may differ from male colleagues in that they are unlikely to have the bonus of a partner who will undertake domestic responsibilities for them, and they will have had to choose between a successful career and children rather than enjoy both, to all intents and purposes they are like men; it is they who have accommodated the employer rather than vice versa. Even then, as Atkinson and Delamont (1990) show with reference to women in the learned professions, the vital acquisition of indeterminate knowledge by a minority group is impaired in highly gendered settings. In any case, there is inevitably a limit to the number of women who choose this option, who opt, in effect, for a career rather than a family, so women's access to the upper echelons of such male-dominated professions, when so structured, will remain modest. Clearly, few children are likely to be socialised in such families, by definition.

Given this pattern, it is clear that training and education systems alone cannot ensure better access for women to areas where currently there are skill shortages. Practices of discrimination against women by employers are an important ingredient in the social processes which perpetuate and recreate segregation in the NITs, as in other male-dominated arenas. And the gender contract which such social processes support lies at the root of gender segregation in employment.

SKILL SHORTAGES IN THE NITs

The concept of skill is conceptually complex and highly gendered: this was discussed in Chapter 5. The power and status of job incumbents have an important impact upon the value put upon the job in question and the extent to which that job is credited with a high skill content. Industrial muscle (through, for example, strong trade union organisation) and gender are crucial signifiers here. In a rigidly segregated workforce, gender thus assumes vital importance in determining the skill component to be attached to a specific job. That perceived skill level is then reflected in the level of pay with which it is rewarded.

Lane (1988) demonstrated the importance of gendering in determining what constitutes higher-level competence in clerical work. As a source of labour for training to fill high-level skill shortages, women secretaries and clerical workers have rich potential, but are entirely overlooked, largely because of their gender. This becomes crucial, as the discussion which follows will illustrate, in the undermining of women secretaries in particular, and in lowering expectations about their capabilities with regard to learning more advanced manipulations of NITs.

Various writers have debated whether labour market changes, such as the expansion of the service sector, the need for 'flexibility' of workers, and the increased development and use of NITs, will lead to deskilling, upskilling, or further polarisation of the skill content of jobs (Ducatel and Miles 1990: 73–75; Gallie 1991). On the whole the support seems to be for the more optimistic view: that is, employees report an increase in their skill level; but there is evidence, too, of polarisation of skills, particularly in the IT and service sectors, and a deeper gender divide as a consequence. This is a complex area, with considerable sectoral and spatial specificities. The point to stress here is the gender dimension: patterns of work organisation adopted by management can affect the skill level of male and female workers in different ways. Technology need not be deterministic: employers have the role of agency in designing patterns of work organisation, and there has been considerable interest in the EU in encouraging worker participation in that design. Part of the mesh of social processes which helps to determine what patterns emerge are attitudes towards women. Managements which hold stereotypical views about the capabilities of women underuse them. Women respond by taking that identity of an unskilled, unvalued person upon themselves: they lose confidence as a result and their lack of ability to learn new technologies becomes a self-fulfilling prophecy.

The NITs allow a rethink on work organisation tied to previous technologies, but they, too, imply a need for different skills for workers, both manual and non-manual, in addition to technical skills. Training for NITs now demands more general skills, such as the capacity to communicate (increasingly this includes proficiency in other languages), an ability to work in teams, diagnostic skills and willingness to take responsibility. These skills are known in Germany as the 'new pedagogics' or social skills (see Rees 1992a).

Some of these skills, such as communication, are often regarded as skills that women excel in, as witnessed by their relative success in personnel management and the caring services. Indeed, communication may emerge as the key social skill. The successful application of NITs is already jeopardised by unintelligible manuals for personal computers and poor communication between engineers, software users and end-users. This is manifested in companies buying expensive, unsuitable equipment that does not meet their specifications, and inordinate amounts of stress and frustration through employees' feelings of lack of control through their inadequate understanding of NITs (Ducatel and Miles 1990: 119). In Germany, training systems now address those elements that are essential to the effective integration of NITs into the workplace, but elsewhere less attention has been paid to these problems, and NITs are still imbued with an exclusively technical ambience.

Rees differentiates between those skills that a vocational and education training (VET) system can produce which comprise technical competences whose content and level matches requirements of employers in general, and those skills which may be wholly specific to an individual firm (Rees 1990: 32). VET systems tend to produce highly transferable skills: in-firm training is more context-specific. The social construction of technical skill depends not just upon which gender performs the task involved, but also on how those skills were obtained. Moreover, skills acquired through education or training are valued and rewarded more than 'talent' thought to be innate or skills learned on the job. Time-served apprentices, however outmoded their skills, are respected and given the highest status in skilled work. Women in low-level IT work tend to acquire their skills by other means, such as 'sitting-by-Nellie' or in-house training: this method of learning skills tends not to be rewarded with a qualification. Moreover, employers sometimes use qualifications as a screening device, a short-cut exclusionary mechanism, rather than identifying them as a requirement for a job in any related sense: young unemployed people during the 1970s and 1980s found that the level of qualifications required for essentially unskilled jobs crept up as the state of the labour market allowed employers to pick and choose.

The issue of skill shortages is, of course, a complex notion depending to an extent on market forces, national societal effects such as culture and institutional structures (Maurice *et al.* 1986) and regional variation. They can be the result of a mismatch between the rate an employer is prepared to pay for skills and that for which a worker is prepared to work. I propose here to summarise some of the most widely identified skill shortages relating to NITs in the EU and to introduce issues surrounding women's access to those jobs. Increasingly, there are shortages of people who combine an understanding of NITs with other skills. This is the case not simply for people, the majority of workers indeed, who increasingly need to use NITs as part of their jobs, but for those in the business of developing and running systems as well. Workers will need to combine an understanding of NITs with the new pedagogics.

The areas of IT already experiencing the most severe shortages, according to Virgo (1991), are as follows:

- highly skilled, state of the art 'technicists';
- 'hybrids' or 'business analysts', who need to be able to understand what new technologies can offer and how to use them; and
- business managers, with responsibilities for recruitment and patterns of work organisation.

These three groups are considered in turn.

Technicists

The current IT 'skills crisis' is largely in high and medium-level IT jobs such as systems programmers, network controllers and application system developers, for which graduate recruitment of people with technical qualifications is the main point of entry. These are what Ducatel and Miles (1990: 156) call the 'industrial heartland IT skills'.

Both Germany and Ireland have specialised in the education and training of such people. The difficulty faced by Ireland has been retaining them: if job opportunities commensurate with their skills are not available locally, they will emigrate to Germany or further afield to countries such as Japan and the US. More recently, however, Ireland has scored some success in attracting these graduates back, their ability to set up profitable companies being enhanced by their European experience and contacts. Even in Germany, however, where there are already job opportunities for people with high-level skills, there are recruitment difficulties, and companies have to address the issue of making jobs attractive enough for the incumbents to want to stay (see Rees 1994b).

Women's access to such high-level NIT employment has been restricted. Where single port of entry systems operate in recruitment to such posts, women's lack of appropriate degree qualifications has traditionally acted as a barrier. Women graduates are clustered in arts and social science subjects and are less likely to have the relevant subject examination passes (for example, mathematics) that would gain them entry to computing and other IT courses at degree level. The lack of routes of progression, both in training systems and in employment between low-level and high-level IT, also acts as an impediment to women's entry. This absence of bridges between subject areas is identified in the EC's White Paper on *Teaching and Learning* as a major problem (see Chapter 9; EC 1996b).

High-level IT work has been characterised by increased credentialism, in other words the demand for qualifications as an entry criterion, and this in part explains the dearth of women in such employment. But even where multi-portal entry systems operate, that is, where it is possible to enter the organisation further down the hierarchy without such qualifications (say, in the middle tiers) and work one's way up through internal promotion, it is noticeable that women who do reach the higher echelons tend overwhelmingly to have gained access through their qualifications, rather than through internal recruitment in what is inevitably a male culture and environment.

The development of NITs may be triggering the shake-up of rigid patterns of segmentation and gender segregation in some sectors such as retailing and financial services, but that does not on the whole apply to IT work itself. The ethos and culture of computing and engineering in particular remain male dominated. Some of the reasons for this, and its effects, are discussed below.

'Hybrids' or 'business analysts'

There is a growth in demand for people to do what used to be called 'hybrid' jobs, which combine business management skills with an understanding of IT: such people are now usually referred to as 'business analysts'. They have an understanding of NITs and possess administrative, strategic and entrepreneurial skills (Ducatel and Miles 1990). The lack of such people has been identified as a main constraint upon the take-up of new technologies in the manufacturing sector in the UK (Christie *et al.* 1990). One major 'core-IT' company emphasised the need for people with general, allround skills, rather than highly specialised IT skills alone, thus:

> A crucial change in our requirements for personnel and their skills is needed for the future. With specific exceptions (such as engineering) we will not need people with specific IT skills. What

we will need are people who can communicate with our customers, interpreting their needs for the system specifiers, who can educate our customers in the benefits of IT and who can appreciate the role of IT generally in the business world. In short, we will be looking for suitable attitudes and a sound broad-based education, not formal skill-based qualifications.

(Seward-Thompson 1987: 25)

The Women into IT Project is a campaign run by major British employers, supported by the Department of Trade and Industry, which seeks to encourage more women to take up opportunities in NITs and to encourage more employers to consider employing women for technical posts. Virgo (1991), from Women into IT, criticises the strategy adopted by many employers (not just in the UK) to fill the shortage of business analysts by converting technical people (of whom there is already a shortage), fuelling further problems in the future. Moreover, people hired for their technical qualifications and skills may not have the personal aptitudes and understanding of business necessary to do the new tasks. They do not universally make a successful transition. NIT skills comprise only part (some commentators have suggested as little as 30 per cent) of the business analyst's job; dealing with people and communication skills are highly important. Nevertheless, the job has become imbued with a 'techie' culture which discourages people who do not regard themselves first and foremost as technical people. The 'techie' culture almost takes a pride in obfuscating the NITs, in effect manipulating discourse to 'own' them and to exclude others, for example through use of language peppered with jargon and sets of initials. An aura of technical sophistication and impenetrability can surround those responsible for managing highly expensive systems. However, business analysts need in essence to *communicate* the benefits of the systems to those who can gain advantage from them; to *share* rather than to possess the technology.

Virgo (1991) argues that, to fill shortages of both technicists and business analysts, recruitment nets need to be widened. The two main obvious groups are non-technical graduates (for example, arts and social science graduates), and existing staff in secretarial and clerical grades. However, secretaries and clerical workers are a grossly under-estimated group: career routes within the organisation for such workers barely exist, and they tend to be overlooked when the firm considers employees to train for higher skills. Both groups are, of course, substantially made up of women. Virgo argues that computing and IT generally have a bad image as far as women are concerned, and that employers, overwhelmingly male, tend not to associate women with such potential skills, nor to recruit them.

Secretaries often provide a 'chauffeured' use of new technology; they 'drive' the technology for their bosses by managing spread-sheets, electronic mail and computerised diaries. Career routes within the organisation for secretaries barely exist. Women arts and social science graduates, however, are unlikely to consider, or be considered for, IT or business analyst posts. Siemens has been successfully retraining unemployed social science graduates in Germany (see Rees 1994b). The social construction of skill hence undermines the appreciation of the potential that women can offer an organisation, but where it makes good business sense, companies can overcome this and train women for skill shortages in these posts.

Business managers

It is essential that business managers appreciate the potential that both NITs and human resources can offer. Without that knowledge and understanding, existing patterns of division of labour are simply superimposed upon new technology, introducing in effect a form of Taylorism in the office, just at the time when it is being superseded in the manufacturing sector. Managers are often not fully aware of the potential that IT has to offer and are unwilling to take the time to be trained themselves – or to admit to the deficiencies a need for training implies. This is particularly the case in the small to medium-size enterprises which employ the majority of the EU's workforce. This is arguably the most difficult skill shortage to address, because there is less willingness to admit that there is a problem, and such enterprises are less likely to have a training budget or culture.

Vickery (1990) identifies a number of issues which are critical to the development of an IT strategy and which hinge on lack of familiarity with the implications and possibilities of IT on the part of business managers. He particularly points to their failure to understand the IT planning process; to cultural barriers between business and IT directors; to problems in the total understanding of database and systems management issues, and in the use of IT effec-tively to deliver customer satisfaction (Vickery 1990: 15).

One consequence of such partial understanding is the persistence of existing gendered patterns of division of labour. In a highly segregated pattern of use, typing pools become data entry or word processing pools, but offer employees reduced job satisfaction. Such deskilled jobs are demotivating, particularly when coupled with poor remuneration, no prospect of advancement and the risk of repetitive strain injury. Moreover, higher expectations of the incumbents of such jobs, because of the new technology (job enlargement rather than job enrichment) can put enormous stress on such workers, particularly when machines are programmed to record numbers of key strokes and targets are set. The powerlessness of workers in jobs designed in this way increases susceptibility to sexual harassment. In such work situations, it is women who lose out, because it is their jobs on the whole which become deskilled. The organisation loses too, however, as there tends to be a fast turnover of staff, so recruitment costs are repeatedly incurred (Fielder and Rees 1991). In a period of labour shortage, such jobs may well be increasingly difficult to fill. Introducing or upgrading IT should ideally involve wholesale job redesign. Training business managers needs to involve not simply alerting them to the potential of new technology for their organisation, but training in de-stereotyping and equal opportunities. Some major international companies have begun to introduce such training for middle and senior management, in the context of staff retention difficulties and skill shortages.

Just as women-only training has proved effective in introducing women returners to new technologies, so some employers have used segregated training for their employees in these fields. Some German high-tech companies where gender segregation is particularly marked have introduced women-only training. Messerschmitt-Bolkow-Blohm, for example, which specialises in high-tech products in the defence and aerospace industry, has women-only training for semi-skilled female workers, secretaries, women in technical and skilled 'male' jobs, and for women returning to the firm (Langkau-Herrmann 1990). AEG offers women-only training in electronics: trainees can enhance their pay and get better jobs within the company, but the company has not gone as far as offering them the opportunity to acquire the full qualification (Rees 1994b). Women-only training for women managers has been used for filling shortages of both business analysts and business managers. Some multinational companies are introducing such training for their female 'high fliers' who can prove to be invaluable for fostering female networks, which in turn may lead to mentors and role models developing.

There is a powerful association between men, machinery and the concept of technical competence: this has been described as the 'masculinisation of technology'. New technology is perceived as young, white, male territory, and this operates as a barrier to the training and recruitment of women and some men. It means that the pool from which people can be recruited to fill skill shortages is circumscribed, and it ensures that both the ethos of NITs, as reflected in computer games, and the use to which they are put, is self-perpetuating.

CONCLUSION

The EC's High Level Expert Group on building an information society recognises the dangers of creating new categories of the excluded, and regards it as essential to avoid this (High Level Expert Group 1996: 32):

> people or groups of excluded people should not be forced to adjust to the new technologies. Rather, the technologies must become more adjusted to human needs.

However, so far the deliberations of the group have not addressed the issue of the gendering of technology. There are chronic skill shortages in NITs in the EU which women should be in a good position to fill. However, the social shaping of technology; the exclusionary mechanisms and the structures of education, training and employment systems, combine to prevent this opportunity from being fulfilled. Indeed, as NITs become more pervasive, women are increasingly likely to be excluded from the benefits, and from determining the design, shape and application of those technologies.

This chapter identifies some of the mechanisms which prevent women from moving into some of the skill shortages in NITs in the EU. The gendering of technology starts at an early age and is reinforced through the experience of computing in school. The use of credentialism to restrict access to higher education and employment in, for example, computing and engineering has meant that subject choices at school made by girls are largely inappropriate for entering these areas. The 'gender-neutral' approach of the EC in its programmes and policies has to an extent reinforced these divisions, although, paradoxically, the EC has also been the main source of funding for many exemplary – if small-scale – women-only projects in new technologies.

VET systems and employers are not geared to the needs of women as parents, as less-qualified individuals, and as strangers in a technological world dominated by men. Women's capacity to fill skill shortages in NITs is impaired by this. At the same time, there will be a greater dependence upon women in the workforce in the future, and the 'new pedagogics' mean that women are ideally suited to fill those skill gaps. There is a clear need, therefore, for policies at a number of levels to bring women and NITs skills shortages together. The next section of this book considers EC education and training policies.

Chapter 7

EC community action programmes on education and training

The European Social Fund, discussed in Chapter 8, is the main instrument through which the European Commission finances training activities in the Member States. However, in 1976 a Resolution of the Council of Ministers indicated that a series of vocational education and training action programmes would also be supported to address particular concerns about the development of human resources. The programmes were designed to target key issues and special groups. They were to be innovative and have a transnational dimension. A series of action programmes was set up in the late 1980s (following Council Decisions) by the Task Force Human Resources, Education, Training and Youth, a sub-directorate of DGV, with the support of a Technical Assistance Office for each one. They included programmes on initial training (PETRA), continuing training (FORCE), student exchange (ERASMUS), the enhancement of advanced technology skills (COMETT) and the development of language competences in the European Community (LINGUA).

In 1991, the French MEP Mme Nicole Fontaine asked a question in the European Parliament concerning equality of opportunity to Community programmes experienced by people of different ages, gender, educational level and 'social category'. The need to respond to this question brought to light the fact that adequate monitoring mechanisms were not in place to furnish the necessary information. An internal report drew together the figures readily available (Bucci 1991). This was followed by further work within the Task Force (Christiansen 1992) for a meeting of the Social Dialogue partners, who were considering the subject of women and training in Madrid in February 1992 in preparation for their subsequent *Joint Opinion on Women and Training* (CEC/Social

Partners 1993) (see Appendix III). It was in this climate of interest in the record of the action programmes on EO that a subsequent, more detailed review conducted by the author (and known as the 'Rees Report' (1995b [1993]) was commissioned by the TFHR later in the same year. The review was based on interviews with key people in the Task Force and TAOs responsible for the programmes, together with an analysis of programme documentation and statistics and both internal and published reports.[1] This chapter draws upon that research to give an account of gender segregation in the programmes and to critique the effectiveness of their equal opportunities (EO) policies.

Reviewing the position of women in the EC's action programmes on education and training in 1992 was particularly timely. There had been increasing concern, both within the Commission and among the Social Partners, about making more effective use of women's potential in the labour force (see Chapter 4). The Community action programmes were scheduled to come to an end in 1994, and the European Parliament had resolved that the EC should review its actions in the field of education and training generally. Plans were being made to extend the competence of the Commission in education and training in the Maastricht Treaty: in the final version, Articles 126 and 127 charged the Commission with the tasks of developing training policy at European level and complementing the activities of the Member States in enhancing quality in education. As a consequence, following the Treaty's coming into effect in 1994, the Commission was able to begin developing guidelines for the design of new Community action programmes in the field of education and training, with an enlarged budget (referred to as the 'Ruberti guidelines', after their author, Commissioner Professor Ruberti) (CEC 1993f). In 1995, the Task Force Human Resources, Education, Training and Youth became a Directorate General in its own right (DGXXII, Education, Training and Youth), and in the same year, all the community action programmes on education and training were replaced by just two new larger programmes, LEONARDO DA VINCI (training) and SOCRATES (education), which incorporated many of the activities of their predecessors.

The principle of equal treatment for men and women, enshrined in the Treaty of Rome, was one of the objectives of all the Community action programmes, as it is of LEONARDO and SOCRATES. But how effective were the policies designed to deliver this objective? To what extent did women benefit from these

Community action programmes, compared with men? And what lessons are there for improving EO in LEONARDO and SOCRATES? This chapter focuses on the programmes up until 1994, and argues that the *laissez-faire* approach to EO which characterised the programmes had the net effect of widening the skills gap between men and women. It concludes that a much more proactive approach needs to be taken. The following chapter examines the approach to EO and the position of women in the first year of LEONARDO and in the ESF. Both chapters seek to address two general questions:

- To what extent can EC programmes be said to be meeting the Single Market's needs for trained women, and women's training needs?
- To what extent is the EO objective being achieved?

The first section of this chapter provides a description of the various action programmes which operated between the late 1980s and early 1990s. There were nine programmes in all, together with a network of women's training projects, IRIS, which was co-funded by DGV (discussed in Chapter 8). Rather than the 'responsive mode' mass funding of the ESF, Community action programmes were by contrast much smaller, and in order to relieve pressure points in the development of the EU's human resources, they focused on specific groups (such as young people) or issues (such as skills in new technologies, continuing training and university/industry cooperation). The programmes achieved a significant level of awareness and participation among the Member States during their lifetime (CEC 1993a).

The second section of the chapter provides a critique of the extent to which the EC, through its guidelines, documentation and mechanisms, actively encouraged applicants and participants of EC training projects to pay attention to EO. It looks at the level of gender awareness in the design of programmes. It examines the extent to which EO is flagged up, or not, through, for example, the wording of programme documentation (Council Decisions, vademecums, guidelines to applicants). Evaluation criteria and monitoring tools are also scrutinised.

The third section reviews women's access to and participation in the programmes (in so far as data allow – their availability or otherwise is in itself a revealing indicator of level of gender awareness). It seeks to assess the impact of the EC programmes as a whole on the training of women. Is the effect transformative; that is, are women's employment prospects qualitatively improved, both in terms of being able to obtain a job, and by securing a job with prospects of further training and promotion? Or do the training opportunities provided merely steer them into low-level, low-skilled, low-paid, 'ghettoised', traditionally female work, with poor terms and conditions of employment? While there are many examples of good practice with regard to training for women within the programmes, the overall approach to EO was found to be haphazard.

The fourth section looks at women-specific projects and initiatives within the programmes, and the final section draws out broad lessons learned from the experiences of the programmes to identify how women's training needs can more adequately be met in the future. In both social justice terms, and as a mechanism to release women's potential to fill skill needs, this chapter shows how the *laissez-faire* approach to EO in EC training programmes is ineffective in developing women's skills. Women's participation in the programmes reflects patterns of inequality in the outside world and further deepens gender segregation in skill levels and the labour market.

DESCRIPTION OF THE PROGRAMMES

The central aims of the Community programmes as specified by the Ministers of Education were identified as follows (CEC 1993a: 2):

- the promotion of closer relations between the education and training systems in Europe;
- increased cooperation between universities and institutions of higher education;
- improved possibilities for academic recognition of diplomas and periods of study;
- encouragement of the freedom of movement of teachers, students and researchers;
- the achievement of equal opportunity for access to education.

To achieve these aims, the TFHR designed programmes which can broadly be described as supporting and developing training throughout the Member States and beyond, in some cases into eastern European and European Free Trade Area (EFTA) countries. This was achieved through instruments which supported networking, mobility and exchange, and transnational projects.

More specifically, Community action programmes provided support for the development of good-quality training tools and methodologies, particularly in the new technologies, fostering transnational networks and exchanges and cooperation between students and teachers, facilitating university/enterprise links, supporting training courses, focusing attention on the need for the training of trainers, and supporting research activities. An overview of the programmes is presented in Table 7.1 (see CEC 1989; 1991c; 1992a; 1993b for more detailed accounts of programmes and activities).

These programmes are now described in a little more detail. Many of the elements now feature in LEONARDO and SOCRATES.

COMETT

In response to the concern of the Council of Ministers to develop technological skills to enhance the competitiveness of the Single Market, COMETT was designed to provide financial support for university–industry cooperation in training for technology. It was geared in particular to advanced technology and the development of highly skilled human resources. The objectives of the programme included supporting projects designed to improve the contribution of advanced technology training to economic and social development, fostering transnational sectoral and regional networks of technology training projects, and responding to the skill needs of small and medium-size enterprises (SMEs). A further objective was to develop a European dimension to cooperation between universities and industry and to initial and continuing training with regard to the application and transfer of technologies. This was tackled through the establishment of regionally based University–Enterprise Training Partnerships (UETPs).

COMETT ran in two phases (1987–89 and 1990–95), and had a number of operational 'Strands' directed at these objectives. Broadly, in the first phase, Strand A comprised the network of UETPs; Strand B was concerned with transnational exchanges for students and personnel; and Strand C was made up of joint projects for continuing training in technology for multimedia distance training. Strand D provided support for promotion and back-up measures. Participation in COMETT was opened to EFTA countries in 1990.

Table 7.1.   Brief description of EC education and training community
action programmes 1986–1994

Scheme	Description
COMETT (1986–95) (206.6 mecu)	Programme on cooperation between universities and industry regarding training in the field of technology
FORCE (1991–94) (31.3 mecu)	Action programme for the development of continuing vocational training in the European Community
PETRA (1988–94) (79.7 mecu)	Action programme for the vocational training of young people and their preparation for adult and working life
ERASMUS (1987–95) (307.5 mecu)	EC action scheme for the mobility of university students
TEMPUS (1990–94) (194 mecu)	Trans-European mobility scheme for university studies
LINGUA (1990–94) (68.6 mecu)	Action programme to promote foreign language competence in the European Community
EUROTECNET (1990–94) (7 mecu)	Action programme to promote innovation in the field of vocational training resulting from technological change in the EC
YOUTH FOR EUROPE (1988–94) (32.2 mecu)	Action Programme for the promotion of youth exchanges in the Community – 'Youth for Europe' programme
IRIS (1988–95) (0.75 mecu)	European network of vocational training projects for women

Notes: 1. Budget details are up to 1992 only. Most of these funds were a 50% contribution matched by the applicants from other sources from their respective Member States; 2. A 'mecu' is a million ecu. An ecu was worth roughly 80p at the time of writing (1996)
Source: Adapted from Commission of the European Communities (1993) *EC Education and Training Programmes 1986–1992. Results and Achievements: An Overview* Luxembourg: Office for Official Publications of the European Communities, COM(93) 151 final, Table 1

FORCE

FORCE was one of the latest programmes to be developed and focused on policy development, innovation and exchange of experience in continuing vocational training. Prompted by the ageing demographic structure of the Community workforce, the EC wanted to support companies seeking to improve the skill levels of existing employees. It concentrated in particular on SMEs, and involved collaboration between trainers and training bodies, public authorities and the Social Partners. Transnational FORCE partnerships and networks comprising these bodies were set up to integrate continuing training into regional development plans and to transfer good practice, especially to the economically weaker regions. A variety of networks, exchange programmes, transnational pilot projects and projects concerned with the evolution of qualifications were funded.

The FORCE TAO was also involved with reviewing continuing training in the Member States through analyses of policies, specific sectors (for example, retailing) and through the examination of collective agreements between employers and trade unions on training (for example, in Italy). Many of the themes of the FORCE programme have reappeared in LEONARDO DA VINCI.

PETRA

PETRA was aimed at young people, a target group identified as warranting particular attention in Community education and training strategy because of high rates of youth unemployment. It grew out of two previous EC action programmes on the transition of young people from school to adult and working life. The first phase included a European Network of Training Partnerships (ENTPs) which focused on joint development and implementation of training modules and the training of trainers. Youth Initiative Projects (YIPs) were managed by young people themselves and sought to provide an alternative learning environment. They aimed to develop an entrepreneurial spirit among young people while developing qualities of assumption of responsibility, self-evaluation, team work and communication skills. Research Partnerships involved transnational research teams exploring key issues in the education and training of young people, such as enterprise.

The second, enlarged and more decentralised phase of PETRA provided a single framework of Community Action in support of vocational training for young people up to and including the age of 27. Action I comprised training and work experience placements in another Member State. Action II was made up of the ENTPs and YIPs of phase 1. Action III consisted of vocational guidance activities, a strong feature of the PETRA programme. A network of national guidance centres was developed. In order to facilitate the free movement of workers within the Single Market, the centres included training for counsellors on the European aspects of vocational guidance among their activities.

ERASMUS

The aim of ERASMUS was to develop closer contact between universities in the European Community and to foster more of a European identity among students. The ERASMUS programme supported student mobility by enabling many more students to spend a recognised period of study in other Member States. The Commission set itself a target whereby 10 per cent of students in the EU should take part in a mobility project of some description. Interuniversity Cooperation Programmes (ICPs) were funded which comprised mobility programmes for students and staff, joint curricular development programmes and short intensive programmes involving students and teachers from several Member States. Teachers and administrators could be funded for study visits, and individuals could apply for short, invited teaching assignments in universities in other Member States. Some other smaller higher education cooperation activities were also funded, such as a pilot scheme for an experimental Community Course Credit Transfer System. EFTA countries have been able to participate in ERASMUS since 1992. ERASMUS activities have been continued under SOCRATES (see Table 7.1).

TEMPUS

TEMPUS (Trans-European Mobility Scheme for University Studies) was set up in reaction to the dramatic political and economic changes in Eastern and Central Europe in 1989 and 1990. The EC was asked by the European Council to design appropriate measures in education and training to support the reform process. The TEMPUS programme was originally aimed at responding to the training needs of Poland and Hungary, but was later extended to other Eastern and Central European countries. It supported various activities available under other action programmes, such as exchange and mobility, particularly for university students, teachers and young people, and cooperation with Member States on training initiatives called Joint European Projects (JEPs). The TEMPUS programme was part of the EC's PHARE (Pologne Hongrie Aide à la Reconstruction Economique) programme of assistance to the countries of Central and Eastern Europe. There are other programmes, too, that seek to develop expertise in Eastern Europe, such as Technical Assistance to the Commonwealth of Independent States and Georgia (TACIS).

LINGUA

LINGUA was designed to develop language communication competence within the European Community. It funded activities supplementary to Member States' own policies in this area. Initial and continuing training of language teachers was supported through, for example, Inter-University Cooperation Programmes. Young people were funded on exchanges under Joint Educational Projects (JEPs). Decentralised actions (managed by the Member States themselves in cooperation with the Commission) included funding teachers and young people to follow courses in countries whose languages they are studying or teaching. Centralised actions (managed by the TAO with cooperation from the Member States) enabled language teacher training centres to join transnational networks to develop new types of language training modules. The issue of language development to facilitate business communication was a particular feature of LINGUA, and these actions more generally have been continued and further developed under SOCRATES.

EUROTECNET

EUROTECNET was one of the first programmes to be established. Its purpose was to promote innovation in the field of initial and continuing training with a view to technological change. It was designed to influence Member State governments in their approach to new technologies.

YOUTH FOR EUROPE

Exchange visits were promoted by YOUTH FOR EUROPE for young people between the ages of 15 and 25 who were not in mainstream education and training. The intention was to foster the development of a new breed of Europeans by exposing young people to first-hand knowledge of other Member States, and helping them to create links and become aware of people from other social backgrounds. A third of the funds was set aside to target young people in geographically remote regions, in which minority languages are spoken. Projects targeting young people from disadvantaged backgrounds were also prioritised.

IRIS

The IRIS network of women's training projects has already been introduced and is clearly of particular interest here. It is, however, a network rather than a programme, and this is reflected in its budget (see Table 7.1). It was set up in 1987 as a response to the Council Recommendation on women's access to vocational training, and was designed to support innovation in vocational training for women. As the IRIS network was originally funded jointly by DGV and the Task Force, it is discussed in the next chapter on structural funds. Funding is only provided for networking activities; it is not supported for training activities as such. The coordination team arrange meetings and conferences, maintain a database of projects and produce bulletins. In 1995 the network became self-financing.

The Task Force identified three main activities as characterising these action programmes (CEC 1993b). These are described below.

Networking   of individuals and organisations to promote exchange of ideas and dissemination of good practice. Networks of various kinds were supported under nearly all the programmes, most notably the 207 COMETT higher education–industry consortia and the ERASMUS and LINGUA interuniversity cooperation projects, in addition to the IRIS network itself.

Mobility and exchange   to promote collaboration. The Task Force estimated that altogether, in the region of a quarter of a million students and trainees, 18,000 young people and 8,500 teachers and training personnel participated in the mobility and exchange programmes (CEC 1993b: 11).

A European dimension   to the content of training, to be promoted by joint transnational projects. The fostering of a European dimension to education and training activities is a particular feature of

FORCE, where the TAO produced synoptic tables on training and qualifications arrangements in the various Member States; and of ERASMUS and COMETT, which, *inter alia*, focus on European strategies within national higher education systems.

To put these activities in context, it should be remembered that the total budget for the Community action programmes on education and training in the period 1987–92 represented only 0.38 per cent of total European Community expenditure, compared with 7.74 per cent spent on the ESF (CEC 1993b: 5). Nevertheless, TAO figures and evaluation reports demonstrate that an impressive level of awareness and participation was achieved across the Member States in these Community action programmes in a relatively short time period. Moreover, the resources were used as a catalyst: the requirement for matching funding in cash or kind from applicants for many of the activities clearly increased the overall amount channelled into projects, while at the same time the EC funds available provided a draw to resources within the Member States.

While the programmes were for the most part evaluated at the levels of project, Member State and programme, the principle of subsidiarity and the fact that many of the activities were networking and awareness-raising activities made their impact difficult to assess, even in broad terms. Evaluation exercises tended also to be limited by lack of available data and the usual restrictions of a *post hoc* approach. EO was clearly identified as one of the five original objectives for the programmes by the Council of Education Ministers, but does not routinely appear as a heading in evaluation reports. To what extent can this objective be said to have been achieved?

The first approach taken in seeking to answer this question is to examine what kind of model of EO is presented in the documentation of the programmes.

EO IN THE EC ACTION PROGRAMMES

The Council of Ministers adopted a Recommendation on Vocational Training for Women in November 1987 which called upon Member States to ensure that:

> women have equal access to all types and levels of vocational training, particularly professions likely to expand in the future

and those in which women have been historically under represented.

(cited in PA Cambridge Economic Consultants 1992: 1)

This section examines whether the provision of EO is clearly specified as an objective in the various training programmes and what model of EO is implied. It also explores the nature of the mechanisms in place to monitor and evaluate the extent to which that objective is achieved. This is assessed through a systematic examination of:

• the wording of the Council Decisions which set up the individual programmes;
• the wording and emphasis in the EO statements in the vademecums and guidelines to applicants for the programmes;
• the wording on application forms specifying what information is required on the gender of target groups;
• the mechanisms and procedures for gender monitoring (for trainees and trainers) for each programme – do they exist, how effective are they for the collection and analysis of statistics, what significance is attached to their accurate collection and verification by different actors?;
• the criteria for programme evaluation and research programmes – to what extent do these pay attention to the issue of EO?;
• the sanctions which are invoked where projects do not seek to provide EO;
• the *animation* (support and development) facilities to encourage and assist projects wanting to develop training for women, or projects with good EO provision;
• the institutional support for EO, for example through TAO staff having EO as part of their portfolio of responsibilities.

We begin by looking at the place of EO in programme objectives.

EO as a programme objective

All the action programmes have an EO statement in the wording of the Council Decisions which set them up, with the exception of that for LINGUA, which did, however, have a commitment to consistency and complementarity with other programmes. By implication this includes EO.

However, there is a significant difference in the wording of the statement between programmes. In some (COMETT, EUROTECNET, FORCE, PETRA), the objective is 'to promote' EO, while in others (ERASMUS, TEMPUS) it is 'to ensure' EO. In English of course, these two terms have significantly different meanings. To 'promote' means to further the growth or development of, while to 'ensure' means to make certain of, to guarantee. However, there are no significant differences in the mechanisms for checking the extent to which EO have been provided between programmes with the two categories of EO statement. Nor was there any discernible difference in the approaches of the programmes apparently offering different levels of commitment to EO.

The second issue here is that of intention. To what extent are EO statements merely intended to ensure that there is no discrimination on the grounds of gender in the legal sense? Or is the intention that people of both genders enjoy effective equality of access? If the latter is the case, their different starting positions need to be recognised and accommodated to encourage equality of outcome.

A third issue relates to the level of energy with which objectives are pursued. If a programme has a small number of well defined objectives, the expectation that they be addressed and indeed achieved may well be greater than if there is a long list of less specific ones. So, if EO is listed among a dozen statements encouraging the participation of specific groups, then its effectiveness may well be lost.

Most of the EO statements describe an equal access model (discussed under the heading of 'equal treatment' in Chapter 3). For example the ERASMUS Council Decision reads ' . . . ensuring equal opportunities for male and female students as regards participation in . . . mobility' (Council Decision, Article (i) (I 1987; II 1989). Some, however, specifically mention women, as in the EUROTECNET Council Decision:

> promoting equal opportunities for men and women, in particular the access of women to types of training with significant technological content, as well as the re-training or re-entry into employment of women, whose professional activities are affected by technological change.
>
> (Council Decision, Article 4.1 (e) 1989)

The extent to which the EO statement as an objective is intended to be taken seriously is indicated by follow-through in vade-mecums and guidelines to applicants. While the COMETT II vade-mecum does contain an EO statement, most applicants' guidelines do not.[2]

Mechanisms of gender monitoring

Gender monitoring mechanisms can be used to examine the gender make-up of programme applicants, project participants, and staff concerned with programme delivery, from the Task Force through to all the delivery agencies. Gender monitoring is an integral part of initiatives which include a commitment to EO. Of those Task Force programmes where it was appropriate, some asked for the gender of applicants and some did not. Of those which did, some TAOs, such as that for ERASMUS, then analysed the data, while most did not.

Ideally, to check for systematic biases, information should be collected on the gender of applicants for trainee and student places on education and training projects which can then be compared with the gender of those accepted. This can allow comparisons between the profile of applicants and that of the successful candidates. Patterns of equality of opportunity and outcome can then be clearly mapped. TEMPUS did this most effectively but the other TAOs did not.

Moreover, participation rates should be looked at in the context of target groups, that is those eligible to participate. For example, although COMETT had relatively few women participating, it had a reasonable 'strike rate' within the eligible target group of trained women. So, for example, the proportion of women engineers participating in COMETT throughout the European Community was higher than the proportion of women among engineering students in higher education in the Member States at the time, as suggested by Eurostat figures.

It is increasingly common practice among large employers in many Member States to use gender (and ethnic origin) monitoring in job application forms in an attempt to limit subconscious discrimination. Information on applicants' gender is collected separately on a form attached to but detachable from the main application. Where appropriate, information on marital status and parenthood (which are associated with gender inequality) can also be collected for monitoring without prejudicing individual applications. Despite the growth in this practice, it is a less widespread part of the recruitment process for students and trainees among mainstream education and training institutions in the Member States, and it did not form part of the monitoring mechanisms requested of projects by the TFHR and the TAOs.

The lack of gender monitoring devices among the education and training action programmes generally made it difficult to assess women's level of participation on a systematic basis.

Programme evaluation and research programmes

To what extent was a gender dimension featured as one of the criteria for programme evaluation and research reports of training programmes? At the time of the review, not all the programmes had been the subject of a publicly available evaluation or annual report. However, an examination of documents available at the time revealed no systematic pattern. Some evaluation criteria certainly did specify attention to EO, for example COMETT (see below). Others, such as LINGUA and ERASMUS, did not. Where an evaluation criterion was specified, the consultants varied in the extent to which they examined the issue: ECOTEC's (1991) evaluation of COMETT did discuss the issue in brief but most reports stopped short of an analysis.

Sanctions and support

On the whole, the stance of the programmes towards EO was a passive one. No sanctions were applied if programmes and projects within them systematically favoured one gender rather than providing a balanced outcome. There is considerable scope for offering encouragement and support to applicants wishing to increase women's participation: some were tried out in the programmes and are a feature of LEONARDO DA VINCI and SOCRATES.

FORCE applicants were asked about the EO dimension of their proposals, and indeed the TAO submitted applications to CREW for further advice. CREW, moreover, accessed the IRIS network to encourage women's training projects to make applications for funding under FORCE.

The gendering of pictorial representations of men and women on programme literature is another method through which messages are conveyed to potential project applicants about EO. As an example, a TAO leaflet about FORCE depicts equal numbers of men and women. However, while the women are in clean white coats, seated at a keyboard or holding test tubes, the men are controlling heavy engineering equipment, ten times their size!

There is a further issue in the message conveyed to applicants through the gender distribution of staff in the hierarchies of the TAOs, UETPs, advisory committees, TFHR and so on. These data are not available, but figures on the distribution of women by grade within the Commission itself reflect standard patterns of vertical gender segregation in major bureaucracies, with few women in Head of Unit posts or above (see EC 1994c).

At the time of the review there did not appear to be any mechanisms in place specifically to encourage and assist projects wanting to develop women-centred activities. However, after the review, when TAOs were specifically asked by the Task Force what initiatives had been developed, a number of innovative support measures were put in place.

In the majority of TAOs no specific member of staff was responsible for the EO dimension of the programme. Where a member of staff could be identified, this responsibility was one of many, and the energies invested in the role varied according to the level of enthusiasm of the individual person. No training was offered to assist the staff in developing this aspect of their work.

This section illustrates that, while EO is flagged up as an objective of the action programmes, mechanisms were not integrated to monitor, report or evaluate the extent to which it had been achieved.

WOMEN'S PARTICIPATION IN THE EC ACTION PROGRAMMES

This section charts the numerical share of education and training opportunities given to women, as statistics allow, on the various programmes. It takes, however, a wider perspective of participation than just numbers. There are evaluative questions to be addressed, such as how does the quality, cost and transformative nature of the training experience of the two genders compare? Do EC training programmes restrict women to traditionally female work? Or do they enable girls and women to move into traditionally male occupations and professions, particularly in those sectors facing skill shortages? How do the programmes perform in terms of ensuring women's access to IT training? How do they relate to women's training needs, and the needs of the EC for women's potential to be developed to fill skill shortages in the Community?

The first point to make here, of course, is that figures are not available for a systematic analysis of women's participation, programme by programme, country by country, so answers to these questions are inevitably partial. From those figures that it was possible to collect, it is clear that, broadly, women's participation in the programmes reflected a *laissez-faire* approach to EO. Participation rates mirrored existing patterns of representation of women in the various target groups (see Table 7.2). PETRA, for example, which is aimed at young people in initial vocational training, shows a balance of the genders (46 per cent of participants in the period 1988–91 were female). However, given there are roughly equal numbers in the target population, this is not surprising. COMETT, by contrast, which is concerned with advanced technology, has a strong bias in favour of men (about two-thirds of participants), although, as mentioned earlier, it compares well with women's participation in the cognate disciplines in education and training systems in the Member States more gener-ally, for example in engineering. COMETT, as Bucci writes (1991: 25), is 'obviously affected by the balance between the sexes of those who are its potential beneficiaries'. Table 7.2 and the following commentary present a summary of the findings (see Rees 1995b for a more detailed account). When analysing gender participation, then, it is important to contextualise in terms of qualifying target groups. However, this may reveal inequalities in the focus of resources on training on target groups which systematically exclude women.

The gender distribution is now discussed programme by programme.

COMETT

Figures on participation by gender were not requested by the TAO until 1989 and no reliable figures were available for COMETT II at the time of the review. Women's participation in COMETT varies by strand and by country, roughly in relation to the proportions of women in the target areas of science, engineering and technology. Bucci (1991) calculates that, overall, roughly two men participated in the programme for every woman. The extremes of country vari-ation are differentials in favour of men of only 2.2 per cent in Spain to a maximum of 70.4 per cent in Belgium. Numerically more significant are the figures of 19.4 per cent in the UK and 42.6 per

Table 7.2.   Women's participation in selected community action
programmes

Programme	% Women
COMETT I (1986–89)	
Strand Ba (Transnational student placements)	34
Strand Bb (Transnational secondments for university and enterprise staff)	15
Strand C (Joint university/enterprise continuing training projects)	20
FORCE (1992)	
Exchange participants	19
PETRA (1988–91)	46
European Network of Training Partnerships (1990)	50
Youth Initiative Projects (1989)	52
Third Joint Exchange Programme	56
Young Worker Exchange Programme (1991)	59
ERASMUS (1990/91)	56
Languages	81
Education	75
Arts	63
Medical Sciences	57
Natural Sciences	42
Engineering	14
TEMPUS (1991/92)	
IMGs (EC to Eastern European countries)	22
IMGs (Eastern European countries to EC)	35

Note: IMGs = Individual Mobility Grants
Source: Compiled from Bucci (1991), Christiansen (1992), O'Brien (1992) and
data supplied by the TAOs

cent in Germany. Interestingly enough, in line with women's much
greater participation in engineering in Eastern European countries,
Christiansen (1992) points out that in Bulgaria there was a 50 per
cent ceiling on women in engineering and a fear was expressed that
they would 'take over'. This underlines the fact that EO concerns
about pattern of gender segregation are culturally specific.

In Strand Ba, of 4,300 students on transnational industrial
placements, 34 per cent were women (O'Brien 1992). They were
more likely to be in management and other areas than in engineering or natural science which comprise the bulk (65 per cent) of
placements. In COMETT I, Strands C and D, women were found to
be more likely to attend a course within their own country than
abroad, and were more likely to come from the university sector
than from enterprises. This is against the overall figure of 72 per

cent of participants coming from enterprises. In 1991, of the 1,170 staff in the regional UETPs in COMETT I, just 421 (36 per cent) were women, the majority at secretarial grades. Only 13 per cent of senior staff and 39 per cent of middle management were women, compared with 90 per cent of secretarial staff (O'Brien 1992).

There were some noteworthy, innovative COMETT projects featuring women (although information about them is not particularly well documented or disseminated), and the TAO sought to enhance the profile of women in its activities. One UETP specialised in women and technology (WITEC); this is discussed below and in Chapter 6.

FORCE

As FORCE was very new at the time of the review (the second round of projects had only just been approved), not many data were available. A number of innovative projects for women were included, such as the AXIA project on women employees' training needs (Rees 1994d). The exchange of teachers and trainers scheme had 19 per cent women in 1992, an increase of 3 per cent on 1991. Of the 83 pilot projects in 1991, 80 specifically mentioned the promotion of EO as one of their five specified objectives from a predetermined list on the application form. However, there is no information available on how these objectives were operationalised, and the implementation of the EO objectives was not examined in the reporting or evaluation procedures.

The FORCE TAO did, however, take a pro-active step on EO by asking CREW to examine proposals and advise upon the feasibility of the EO objectives where these had been specified. It was also one of the few programmes which kept figures on the gender of key participants such as project contractants (those entering into the formal contract on behalf of their institution) and project coordinators. The data show that women did not feature strongly among either, as Table 7.3 demonstrates.

Women comprised 19 per cent of participants in the exchanges in 1992. Of these, 7 per cent (3 per cent in 1991) were staff representatives; 16 per cent (8 per cent) were from the Social Partners; 53 per cent (61 per cent) were trainers; and 24 per cent (29 per cent) directors of human resources (1991 figures in brackets).

Table 7.3.   FORCE project contractants and coordinators, 1991 and
1992

	Proportion of women		
	Exchanges No. (%)	Pilots No. (%)	Qualifications No. (%)
	1991 (165 projects)		
Women contractants	4 (1.5%)	8 (4.8%)	2 (1.2%)
Women coordinators	12 (7.2%)	16 (9.7%)	3 (1.8%)
	1992 (260 projects)		
Women contractants	1 (0.4%)	14 (5.3%)	5 (1.9%)
Women coordinators	6 (2.4%)	29 (11.1%)	16 (6.1%)

PETRA

The TAO had to rely on National Grant Awarding Authorities (NGAAs) for data on participation in projects by gender. As PETRA is an initial training-based programme, one would expect a relatively high female participation. And indeed we find that, for the period 1988–91, 39,000 young people aged 15–25 were involved with PETRA, of whom 18,000 (46 per cent) were young women. Half the participants in the ENTPs were women (1990), as were 52 per cent of those involved in the Youth Initiative Projects (1989) (PETRA TAO). Overall female participation on work experience and training periods abroad for young workers or unemployed on the Third Joint Exchange Programme was 56 per cent (Bucci 1991).

Increasing the participation of girls and young women was identified as a main theme for the ENTPs in 1991, and mentioned as a transversal theme in 1988, 1990 and 1992. However, only 66 out of 500 (13 per cent) projects chose to work on this theme, and the majority of these were in schools or colleges, training centres or local/regional authorities rather than employment centres or social partner based. The three main foci were technical education/vocational training courses on trade and crafts, commercial and office administration, and services trades and tourism.

A survey in 1990 of the 1989 Youth Initiative Projects indicated that, of the 2,500 young people involved in the management and development of the projects, 48 per cent were women. About 50 of the 600 projects supported between 1988 and 1992 worked explicitly with young women or focused their activities on women (Banks 1992). EO was not identified as a theme in the research strand. However, more than half the research partnerships started in 1991 were run by female project leaders.

There are striking country and regional differences in all these components. PETRA was also characterised by a traditional pattern of young women comprising the majority of service sector placements, and young men the majority in more technical placements.

ERASMUS

The ERASMUS TAO has already been identified as one which both collected and analysed data on the gender of participants, students and staff. The selection of students is made by participating universities and individual network coordinators. Information on the sex of the applicant is collected on the application form, and records are maintained on the sex composition of grant recipients (students and staff). The TAO then conducts analyses of gender distribution by subject and country.

The female proportion of university students taking part in ERASMUS gradually increased over the years until a roughly equal balance of sexes was achieved. This is one of the programmes where female participation is greatest, and indeed is slightly higher than that of males. Given that the majority of university students are in their late teens or early twenties, these women tend not to be as constrained by domestic commitments as women who might seek to participate in continuing training programmes.

However, although the numbers of participants are about equal, the distribution across the subject spectrum follows traditional lines and has remained more or less constant over the years. Hence, there is a high female participation in languages, education and the arts, and low participation in engineering. Natural and medical sciences are more evenly balanced. Women were least represented in engineering, mathematics, and geography and geology.

The participation of female staff in visits rose from 21 per cent in 1989/90 to 31 per cent in 1992/93. Women are well represented in the NGAAs but poorly represented on Academic Advisory Groups, the ERASMUS Advisory Committee and among the ICPs' management. In the ICPs, women comprise less than 50 per cent of female directors, even in those subject areas where women students are most numerous.

TEMPUS

This action programme was not set up until September 1990. It includes Joint European Projects (JEPs) for the development of teaching capacities at higher education institutions (including cooperative projects with industry and enterprises); Individual Mobility Grants (IMGs) for both students and teachers in higher education; and measures complementary to these two, such as surveys and studies.

TEMPUS has among the best data on gender of all Task Force programmes on the IMGs. IMGs are available from EC countries and from those eligible countries from Eastern Europe (Bulgaria, Czechoslovakia, Hungary, Poland, Romania, Yugoslavia). TEMPUS collects the information on all applicants, and compares it with successful applicants, so that the success rate for each gender can be calculated.

There is a striking difference between the proportion of women among the EC IMG recipients and those from Eastern European countries eligible to participate (see Table 7.2). In 1992, women made up 27 per cent of European Community IMG participants but 35 per cent of those from eligible Eastern European countries. Participation rates of women from the EEC to the eligible countries was 22 per cent compared with 35 per cent in the opposite direction. The advantage in monitoring applications is revealed in the finding that, in EEC countries, women made up only 21 per cent of applicants, whereas in eligible Eastern European countries, the figure was 40 per cent. The relatively small numbers of female participants from Member States is undoubtedly in part because members of the target group are likely to have school-age children, and it is exceedingly difficult either to leave them or to take them. With regard to Eastern European countries in particular, the EC is merely financing and administering the programme; it is up to the individual countries to decide which projects and individuals they want to participate.

Women are thought to be employed in significant numbers in the NGAAs in the eligible Eastern European countries. An interesting observation by a member of the TEMPUS TAO is that this may be both because of their linguistic abilities and because many new governments (for example that of Poland) have been anxious to recruit people with 'clean' political backgrounds and have therefore recruited sociologists (who tend disproportionately to be women in many Eastern European countries), because of the 'non-communist content' of the discipline.

LINGUA

Unfortunately, systematic figures on the breakdown of participation by gender are not available for LINGUA. However, as one would expect in a language-based programme, given the relatively high rates of participation by women on language courses more generally, a rather higher female participation rate is found in LINGUA than in some of the other programmes. Among the decentralised actions (that is, where allocation decisions are made within the Member State rather than by the Commission or the TAO), such as the exchange of 16 to 25-year-olds, women's participation is thought by the TAO to be high, reflecting the picture in the institutions involved. Action 1B, the European Cooperation Programme, provides for networking between institutions and in-service training of teachers. Of course, as teaching is a highly feminised profession, so female participation rates are high.

LINGUA contracts with institutions rather than individuals, and so responsibility for selecting participants is one stage removed: this issue of subsidiarity (to which we return later) is clearly crucial in reflecting cultural patterns within Member States and their institutions. Also, much of LINGUA's work is concerned with the development of didactic materials; it would require a very different kind of analysis to assess their gender dimension.

EUROTECNET

Designed to promote innovation in the field of initial and continuing training with a view to technological change, EUROTECNET was intended to influence Member State governments in their approach to new technologies. It was largely concerned with the development of materials (see EC 1995c for details of a compendium).

This section has focused on women's participation in EC training projects. It shows that, due to lack of systematic collection of statistics by the programmes, our knowledge of the pattern of participation must remain partial. However, even if perfect data were available, this would not help us to gauge men's and women's relative *quality* of experience on the various programmes, in terms of skill enhancement. Nor would it help us to measure the EC's value for money in terms of return on investment through the transformative value of training. That would need a much more thoroughgoing analysis, with proper performance indicators and monitoring instruments.

Overall, however, it is clear from these figures that female participation in EC training programmes is, predictably enough, a reflection of women's participation in the arenas that are targeted. Of most concern is the low level of participation in the technologically oriented programmes, except in specific ringfenced projects that constitute a very small minority of 'showpiece' projects (discussed below). Women appear in much larger numbers in the educationally-based exchange schemes which, while valuable, are not likely to be as transformative in nature. In short, despite equality of opportunity, equality of outcome is far from ensured; rather, patterns of participation reinforce the *status quo*.

WOMEN-SPECIFIC PROJECTS

Of all the action programmes, only the IRIS network focused exclusively on women. However, there were various initiatives and projects within other programmes that were directed at women and some were quite effective in challenging arenas such as training women in large male-dominated enterprises or in advanced new technologies. This section highlights a few of these projects and structural supports built into the programmes where they existed.

Under the COMETT Programme, one UETP, rather than being regionally-based like all the others, was designed to assist at a European level on advising on how to support women wanting to develop technological skills where there are chronic skill shortages (discussed in Chapter 6). The Women into Technology UETP (WITEC) was based at the University of Sheffield in the UK and had a remit to offer COMETT and the other UETPs advice, information and support generally on women and technology. It provided information and data, ran workshops and distributes a newsletter. It played an active role in alerting the TAOs and the other UETPs to issues relating to women and technology. In addition, individual projects within FORCE and COMETT were specifically aimed at women, and, of about 300 demonstration projects in EUROTECNET, 15 (around 5 per cent) were described as being aimed wholly or mainly at women.

A few other UETPs had an overt focus on women in their activities or in specific projects, such as FEAT/ICT Formación de Formadores en Ambitos Técnologicos in Barcelona, and GATEWAY EUROPE in Wales which coordinated the ATHENA and AXIA projects.

EO is included as a subject area under Education and Social Science in the ERASMUS programme. Several networks focused on the broad approach to EO (including anti-racism, social justice, democracy, and human rights) and five exclusively on Women's Studies. Funding has been given to promote excellence and develop the curriculum in Women's Studies in the framework of supplementary measures. This is being continued under SOCRATES.

CONCLUSION

This chapter has reviewed the approach taken to EO in the EC's action programmes on education and training position, and has examined the pattern of participation of women in those programmes in so far as data allowed. The absence of gender monitoring was a finding in itself. Better project documentation would have allowed a more thoroughgoing analysis of the nature of the curriculum, methods of selection and recruitment, the ideology underlying the various projects and so on. However, even with the limitations of the approach that it was possible to take, it is clear that the net effect of the programmes is to reinforce the *status quo*. Men have better access to the more expensive, technical, transformative training; women appear in equal numbers only in school or initial training exchanges and are in the majority only in language-based student mobility programmes such as ERASMUS. The programmes, rather than effecting change, reflect existing gender divisions.

The extent to which women participate in equal numbers varies enormously by country, region, programme, sector, size of establishment, and age group. The variation is not random. EO policies need to take on board the inequalities that exist in the societies they address. Reactive policies can reinforce the *status quo* and lead to further polarisation.

The equal treatment approach to EO, then, which characterised the programmes, proved to be limited in its impact. Positive action projects within the programmes, while highly effective in developing the skills of the relatively small number of women who had access to them, did not affect mainstream provision. The experience of the Community action programmes suggests that, in order to make a significant difference to women's skill levels, it is necessary to reorient mainstream education and training provision, placing women's needs at centre stage. To be effective, much stronger mechanisms are required to assist the programmes to swim against the tide of institutional structures and cultural biases, patterns and attitudes which mean that, in effect, women are much less likely to benefit significantly from the programmes than are men.

The framework of EO outlined in Chapter 3 comprised policies which 'tinker' with EO by addressing the issue in documentation and by carrying out gender monitoring; those which 'tailor' existing schemes to orient them a little more towards the needs of women, to 'build women in' more effectively or address their 'special needs'; and those which 'transform' the programmes much more overtly, 'mainstreaming' some of the lessons learnt from best practice. In essence, the last of these approaches, mainstreaming, seeks to tackle the difficult task of designing programmes which prioritise women's training needs as an objective (in addition to, rather than in exclusion of, the current unrecognised prioritisation of those of men). Of these strategies, ranging in duration from the short to the long term, it is the longer-term strategy which has the capacity to be transformative (rather than reflecting the outside world), and to meet the skill needs of the EU. It is also clearly the most challenging and difficult to achieve.

The programmes described in this chapter came to an end in 1994/95, although most of the activities were continued in the two new, simplified programmes which replaced them, LEONARDO DA VINCI and SOCRATES. The position of women and the approach taken to EO in LEONARDO and in the ESF are the subject of the next chapter.

Chapter 8

The European Social Fund and LEONARDO DA VINCI

Spring is in the air, which means it is the season for looking for partners. There is a flurry of transnational companion-seeking for EC-funded LEONARDO DA VINCI training projects through all the usual outlets: promoters' events, contact fairs and e-mail databases. At the various 'contact fairs', notice-boards are plastered with requests from people desperate for partners with particular attributes: 'Italian women's training workshop on construction skills seeks Finnish partner, please leave a business card in this envelope to say where we can meet'; 'Danish new technology project is looking for a Greek partner, please phone this number'; 'I am the director of a further education college in England looking for partners from Belgium and Portugal for a pilot project on learning disabilities: please meet me in the hotel bar at 6 o'clock if you are interested'. Partners from new Member States are much in demand as it is believed this will increase the likelihood of being funded. Equally, partners from southern countries are at a premium, particularly if they have language skills. Newcomers to the transnational scene are looking for experienced partners. Everyone wants reliable partners who are multi-lingual. Those based in desirable locations seem particularly popular. The discourse of partner-seeking is inevitably reminiscent of the personal ads in the newspaper: 'single mature bachelor with GSOH seeks NS woman interested in theatre, with view to friendship, and maybe more'. LEONARDO DA VINCI, the EC's action programme for training, could be described as acting as an enormous dating agency for European training bodies.

LEONARDO DA VINCI and (if I may call it that) its sister action programme on education, SOCRATES, were introduced by the European Commission (EC) in response to its new competences enshrined in the Maastricht Treaty (Articles 126 and 127). These are to develop a European level strategy for training and education to complement the work of Member States. The Commission's White Paper, *Teaching and Learning: Towards a Learning Society* (EC 1996a), identifies the development of a skilled workforce as vital to the goals of creating jobs, combating unemployment and avoiding social exclusion. These are themes that feature strongly in the other two major White Papers, on economic (1994a) and social policy (1994b), which set the framework for the development of the EU into the next millennium.[1] A flexible, skilled workforce committed to lifelong learning is seen as crucial for the future economic competitiveness of the Single Market. This is rather an ambitious attempt to create a paradigm shift in people's orientation towards learning. To focus attention on this, 1996 was declared the Year of Lifelong Learning, which gave rise to a range of conferences, events and workshops, not to mention column metres of press coverage throughout the EU and a rather nice logo where, as more light shone on a sequence of round faces, their smiles increased in radiance.

LEONARDO DA VINCI as an action programme has been designed by the Commission to tackle specific areas which have been identified as needing special attention in the development of a learning society. The budget is relatively modest and the intention is that it should be used to develop innovative approaches and training materials, many of which are in an electronic format (see EC 1996d, 1996e). The programme also seeks to create an opportunity for transnational learning through pilot projects and the exchange of training providers, students, trainers and trainees. Ideally, if a new method or training material is developed successfully, it should then be disseminated and become embedded in existing practices and provision.

For most of the 'Strands' of LEONARDO (see below), applicants can apply direct to the Commission for financial support. This is in contrast to the procedure for applying for Structural Funds (described in Chapter 4), where Member States themselves apply for funding from the EC. The Structural Funds are made up of the European Regional Development Fund (ERDF); the European Agricultural Guidance and Guarantee Fund (EAGGF), the Financial Instrument for Fisheries Guidance and the somewhat curiously misnamed European Social Fund (ESF). The aim of the Social Fund is to improve employability, mainly through economic development and vocational training. It is the ESF and

LEONARDO DA VINCI and their approaches to EO which are the focus of this chapter.

In so far as data allow, the chapter looks specifically at the position of women within the ESF and LEONARDO. It argues that, just as we have seen in Chapter 7 with regard to the previous EC action programmes (the forerunners of LEONARDO and SOCRATES), and in Chapter 4, with regard to the EC and EO more generally, it is possible to trace a shift in approach from equal treatment through positive action to the current doctrine of mainstreaming equality. These two EC mechanisms for supporting training and the developing human resources are very different: ESF is financially much more substantial than LEONARDO, but involves competition between the Member States. LEONARDO is intended to be used strategically to address 'pressure points' and encourage the development of transnational approaches towards fostering innovation. Both have the capacity to lever 'matching' funding. The broad question being addressed is, to what extent does the existence of these programmes reinforce, challenge or reproduce the gendered segregation of training in the EU?

THE EUROPEAN SOCIAL FUND

The ESF was first set up in the Treaty of Rome, and there is a legal commitment to the equal treatment of men and women within its activities. Its focus has moved through a series of phases since 1957, reflecting shifts in labour market policy which, in turn, are informed by a reading of economic and social change.

There are various formulations of the stages (see, for example, Brine 1995b; Neave 1990; Rainbird 1993). Brine (1995b) identifies four phases, the first running from the late 1950s to the mid-1970s, during which the primary concern was cyclical youth unemployment. During the second, from the late 1970s to the mid-1980s, the attention began to shift to structural unemployment. The third period Brine describes, from the mid-1980s to 1993, saw shifts in the role of vocational education and training. This was manifested in both a 'vertical extension of vocational policy' (Brine 1995b: 149) within Member States, and an increasing tendency towards the vocationalisation of education. She then identifies a fourth period, beginning in 1994, where the administrative and policy linkages between education, training and the economy were further strengthened.

These four phases do reflect the activities of the Member States and the use made of the ESF, although my own view is that it took well into the early 1980s before it was widely accepted that sustained high rates of youth unemployment were the outcome of structural rather than cyclical factors. Rates of youth unemployment were particularly high in the early 1970s due to a convergence of demographic, recessional and other economic factors (notably the oil crisis), together with patterns of restructuring which decimated youth labour markets. This gave rise to a 'moral panic' about the out-of-work young people becoming disengaged from society (Mungham 1982). Indeed, the language of the Schwartz (1981) report on the integration of young people into society and working life in France, commissioned by the French Prime Minister in 1981, is very redolent of the discourse of social exclusion in the 1990s. In the late 1970s and early 1980s, it was increasingly recognised with some alarm that youth unemployment was not exclusively the preserve of the disadvantaged or marginalised (see Neave 1990). The concern was reflected in the late 1970s and early 1980s in a series of job creation programmes in the Member States, many of which were substantially underwritten by the ESF. Young people were particularly targeted (see Rees *et al.* 1980 and Rees 1980, 1983 for an evaluation of such schemes in Eire and Northern Ireland).

The moral panic about youth unemployment in the 1970s, which drove many of the policy responses, was focused almost entirely upon young men. There was especial concern that they would turn to crime and violence if they did not have an opportunity to make the transition to employment, and thereby have an investment in the established order. A job, and the income, status and relative independence one accrued, were marks of adulthood. Without it, young men needed to establish their adulthood in alternative ways.

This conceptualisation was particularly evident in discussions about Northern Ireland, where rates of youth unemployment were higher than anywhere else in the EU and where there was a particular concern about young unemployed men being recruited into paramilitary organisations (Rees 1983). For example, Members of Parliament in the UK saw the 'problem' in the following terms:

Mr Kenneth Lewis: I am sure that the Minister is aware that when young men cannot get jobs, especially in the circumstances existing in Northern Ireland, they become involved in violent mischief. When they obtain dead-end jobs, they become involved in moonlighting and violence. Is he aware that, according to my information, the opportunities in Northern Ireland for young men to become trained in skills are inadequate?

(Hansard 5 July 1979)

Mr James Prior: Among the young unemployment is very high and that is an encouragement to men of violence to attract young people to their ranks.

(Hansard 28 April 1982)

Overall, young women made up only a third of participants in the various schemes supported by the ESF in the early 1980s in Northern Ireland (Rees 1983). They predominated in the (relatively few) schemes for the less able school-leavers, and in the cheaper schemes, such as the Work Experience Programme. Young men, by contrast, were found in the high-quality schemes which offered recognised and sustained training, and a route to the labour market.

Enterprise Ulster, the EU's (then) longest-running job creation scheme for adults, which targeted the long-term unemployed and provided them with training and experience until they found a job however long it took, and which was co-financed by the ESF, only offered places to men. Women who worked for the organisation in an administrative capacity were featured as 'pin-ups' in the house-journal *EU Forum*. Examples of photograph captions included:

Pat Garret, Finance's friendly personality gives a welcome change in statistics . . .

(*EU Forum* Autumn 1979: 1)

Personnel Pin-up Pauline McGrath, our Page One Girl.

(*EU Forum* June 1979: 1)

when Dora Robinson called in to visit the men at the Old Warren play area site in Lisburn, there was no shortage of instructors to show her how the cement mixer works.

(*EU Forum* June 1977: 1)

Gender was a highly significant factor in who was offered what opportunities in ESF-supported schemes in Northern Ireland, and provision was shaped by the social construction of a moral panic about the disorder that unemployed men compared with workless women would create. The main concern about young unemployed women was usually couched in fears about their becoming young single parents, or falling into prostitution (see Mungham 1982). This is redolent of the demonisation of young single mothers on the

St Mellons housing estate in Cardiff by the (then) Secretary of State for Wales, the Rt Hon John Redwood, in 1995. Despite these fears about young women, they were not regarded in the 1970s and 1980s as sufficiently damaging to the moral order for significant steps to be taken to address female unemployment through the ESF.

A series of pilot projects was set up throughout the (then) Member States, funded through the EC's Education to Working Life Programmes, during the 1970s and early 1980s.[2] The documentation for these programmes is not as detailed as the current European programmes, so our information about their impact on young women is limited. Nevertheless, IFAPLAN, the social research institute based in Cologne, charged by the EC with the responsibility for coordinating the programme, commissioned a *post hoc* study to examine the position of women in the projects. The results revealed a lack of gender monitoring statistics. The study also showed the familiar story whereby the 'equal treatment' approach to EO led to young women being among the minority of participants, and to clear gender stereotyping in training and other activities (Rees and Varlaam 1983).

In the late 1980s and early 1990s, Structural Funds were used less for the job creation schemes and more for training. This began the thrust to link education closer to the 'needs' of the labour market and to develop vocational education policies. The focus was less exclusively on special projects for particular disadvantaged target groups (although these remain and, indeed, funding for them has been extended) and more on restructuring education and training systems to facilitate the development of a skilled workforce. Some of the measures in LEONARDO are geared precisely to the development of good practice in order to impact upon systems within the Member States.

A landmark in this rethinking of an approach to training and unemployment was the document known as the Ruberti guidelines (CEC 1993f), Professor Ruberti being the (Italian) EC Commissioner responsible for Education. The document not only set out the structure for LEONARDO and SOCRATES but also influenced reforms to the Structural Funds. This put a much greater focus on training as a human resources strategy in the context of the Single Market, and the development of a 'European dimension' to education. The economic and social purposes of vocational education are brought together. The concern with disadvantaged groups continues, but education and training are also seen as important in their own right to develop a competitive economy. These themes, which feature strongly in the Ruberti document, can be traced through to the economic, social and teaching and learning White Papers (see Chapter 9).

Equal treatment? The position of women in the ESF

One of the most powerful attributes of the Structural Funds is that national governments within the Member States are encouraged to develop projects in order to lever funds from Europe. By the same token, organisations within the Member States can make a case for accessing funds from their own national, regional or local governments through the prospect of attracting matching funds from the EC. The Community Objectives, agreed by the Council of Ministers, which shape the direction for funding are therefore crucial. They are set out in Table 8.1.

To enable Member States to design projects to address these Objectives, the Commission draws up Community Support Framework (CSF) documents, setting out its approach. Member States make bids to the EC by drawing up a series of Operational Programmes (OPs) in response to the strategy and rationale for distribution of funds laid down in the CSFs.

Women are eligible under all the Objectives. In addition, a small

Table 8.1.   Structural Funds: Community Objectives

Community objectives	
1	To promote the development and structural adjustment of regions whose development is lagging behind
2	To convert regions seriously affected by industrial decline
3	To combat unemployment and to facilitate the integration of young people
4	To facilitate the adaptation of workers to industrial change and to changes in production
5a	To speed up the adjustment of agricultural structures
5b	To promote the development of rural areas

Notes: 1. Only the EAGGF takes action under Objective 5b; 2. Regions whose *per capita* GDP is less than or close to 75% of the Community average are classified under Objective 1: this amounts to about 26.6% of the total population budget has been earmarked for projects under Objectives 3 and 4 CSFs in regions not covered by Objective 1. These are aimed at women, as a 'disadvantaged group', alongside other dedicated funds for groups such as migrants and the disabled.

Initiatives from the Member States account for the vast majority of spending under the Structural Funds. However, some 9 per cent of the budget is set aside for Community Initiatives, to fulfil specific aims that fall under the broad Objectives, such as area regeneration or the development of human resources. For example, projects to stimulate employment can be supported in rural areas (LEADER), in urban areas (URBAN), and in regions which were heavily dependent upon defence industries (KONVER), shipbuilding (RENAVAL), steel production (RESIDER), coalmining (RECHAR) and textiles (RETEX). The EMPLOYMENT initiative, launched in 1995 and due to end in 1999, is aimed at developing human resources and is targeted at disadvantaged groups. It is made up of four strands: NOW (New Opportunities for Women), discussed later in this chapter; HORIZON, for the disabled; Youthstart, for young people; and most recently, INTEGRA, aimed at the EU's most disadvantaged, such as travellers, ex-offenders, the long-term unemployed and people with alcohol-related problems. ADAPT and ADAPT-BIS comprise another Community Initiative, this time aimed at those under threat of redundancy as a result of industrial change.

The Structural Funds have a budget considerably larger than that of LEONARDO: for the period 1989–93, the ESF budget alone came to 20,792 billion ecu (Eurostat 1996: 97). One of the difficulties in trying to assess what proportion of this went to women, and the more general impact of the ESF on women, is the lack of gender monitoring. Lefebvre (1993) makes this point in relation to ESF co-financed measures in a report which draws upon a series of individual country studies commissioned by the EC. She concludes that the statistical base is poor throughout the EU. The research teams for the individual Member States had to rely on what information they could glean from data sources such as application forms and annual reports by national and regional authorities.[3] Just like the review of women's position in the TFHR action programmes on education and training, described in Chapter 7, it became clear that gender monitoring is not a significant element in the administration of Structural Funds at the regional, national or European level.

Despite these difficulties, Eurostat provide annual estimates of the gender breakdown of ESF beneficiaries, the most recent of which suggests that 42 per cent of participants are female, a slight increase on previous years (Eurostat 1996). This figure disguises wide country variations, however. In Denmark and Greece, women are the majority of participants, whereas in France, 86 per cent of recipients are thought to be men (Eurostat 1996: 104). Portugal has the highest proportion of participants relative to its population (male and female combined), whereas the UK has the largest absolute number of beneficiaries (3.5 million people), nearly 70 per cent of whom are long-term unemployed. It will be remembered that the UK is one of very few Member States where recorded male unemployment (including long-term unemployment) is higher than that of women. This is due to the fact that many older married women (who have historically paid the 'married woman's stamp' for National Insurance), and women wanting to work part-time, fail to satisfy the eligibility criteria for the JSA. This means that, in the Member State with the largest number of ESF beneficiaries, the majority are always likely to be men.

While Eurostat can provide broad figures, their validity is uncertain, and no explanation is provided for the significant country variations in participation by gender. To what extent do the various Member States identify women's training needs as a priority within their OPs? Brine (1992: 155) shows in her analysis from the early 1990s that:

> All member States, except Italy, prioritised objective 3 (unemployed adults aged over 25), over objective 4 (unemployed people aged under 25) and all the member States, except Luxembourg, specified women in both objectives; the majority showed women as their number 3 priority. The exceptions to this general consensus are Germany, who show women as a priority 1 in both objectives; Italy who give women the lowest priority in both objectives, and Luxembourg, who mention women first in objective 3, and not at all in objective 4.

Given that women have higher rates of unemployment than men, including long-term unemployment, and that they comprise the majority of the low-skilled and disadvantaged workers in the EU, the fact that they are not at the top of the Member States' priority lists, nor the majority of ESF beneficiaries, is clearly a paradox.

Gender segregation within ESF co-funded measures is also an

issue. Lefebvre (1993) found that such schemes tended to reproduce the sexual divisions of the employment market (again echoing the finding in the review of TFHR action programmes, where participation patterns reflected the gender make-up of the target groups). She argues:

> It all goes to show that ESF co-financed measures may well be open to men and women in theory, but they are neither neutral or asexual in practice and they reproduce the discriminations of the employment market. It would take more than bumping up the numbers of women involved in general measures to do away with this discrimination, just as it would take more than bumping up women's employment rates to do away with the division between the traditionally male and traditionally female sectors.
>
> (Lefebvre 1993: 20)

Brine (1992) provides some support for this view in her examination of the influence of the ESF on the vocational training of unemployed women in the UK. She argues that applications for one type of training are prioritised over others, with the net effect that women are steered towards training and employment in male manual jobs in declining sectors, instead of either advancement in traditional female sectors or in new technologies. This is a result of focusing on training women with particular difficulties in the labour market (often through a combination of class and race disadvantages) in areas where they are under-represented. By contrast, developing their skills, and those of other women in new technologies or in advanced female-dominated areas, would make their occupational mobility much more likely.

Lefebvre (1993) notes that there is a mismatch between those most in need and those who participate. The figures show that, with the exception of Denmark and Italy, the percentage of female beneficiaries declines as the level of qualifications rises:

> The majority of women are thought to start out with the wrong qualifications or no qualifications at all and end up with a basic qualification. But a larger percentage of men with no qualifications at the outset end up with medium-grade qualifications.
>
> (Lefebvre 1993: 21)

Lefebvre claims that, on the positive side, all Member States have integrated the equal treatment concept into their legislation and policies on employment and training and have set up special agencies responsible for EO. However, without a more detailed gendered breakdown of kind of activity, it is difficult to tell whether the effects of ESF are closing the skill gap, or widening it, like the early TFHR action programmes described in the previous chapter.

This section shows the haphazard and variable approach to equal opportunities and to women's training across the Member States. Moreover, equal treatment clearly does not produce equal outcome. What spaces are there within ESF for women's projects?

Positive action

At various stages in its history, part of the ESF budget has been earmarked for women's projects. In the period 1989–93 for example, 5 per cent of ESF resources (380 mecu) were used for schemes specifically targeted at women (Eurostat 1996). Whitting and Quinn (1989) make a strong argument in support of naming women as a priority and reflecting this in the allocation of specific funds because it encourages the development of local labour market strategies that address gender, and thereby make the circumstances and needs of women more visible.

Certainly the identification of specific resources to meet women's training needs may prompt the making available of matching funds which might not otherwise have been so allocated. The ESF has acted as a catalyst to the development of women's training projects in the UK simply by enabling training providers, such as women's workshops for example, to operate the ESF lever (Rees 1992b). Indeed, this facility has arguably led to the expansion of third-sector providers in many parts of the EU, whose main source of income comprises European funds 'matched' by local and regional authorities.

Individual Member States have their own organisations, usually in the voluntary sector, that focus on women's training and act both as national-level networks, lobbyists and sources of information and expertise (see Lefebvre 1993). In the UK, the *Women's Training Network* and *Women in Manual Trades* fulfil some of these functions. NIACE, the National Organisation for Adult Learning, holds events on adult education and training for women (see also NIACE 1996). In France, *Racine* is a state-funded, national centre of expertise on Community programmes. *Retravailler* is a major provider of training courses for women returners in France which has now extended its activities to address the needs of other disadvantaged groups. In other Member States, too, the significance of training to the culture can be read off from the existence of sizeable national institutions which regulate, research and document training and contribute to the development of training policy debates. These include the Bundesinstitut für Berufsbildung (BIBB) in Germany, and ISFOL, a centre for the development of vocational training for workers in Italy. Both conduct major research projects on training. Some, such as BIBB, are state funded, others are private organisations which receive some funding from the state. However, significantly, over the last decade, these organisations have developed transnational lines of communication, in part at least as a consequence of the activities of the IRIS network.

The IRIS network, which has been referred to in previous chapters, arose as a consequence of the 1987 EC *Recommendation on Vocational Training for Women* (CEC 1987b), which emphasised the need for women to have access to training in all employment categories where they are under-represented. Initially funded by the EC (DGV and the TFHR – now DGXXII – combined), and based in Brussels, the network soon grew to service nearly 500 women's training projects. It was coordinated first of all by CREW, an independent women's cooperative; a consortium of organisations (including CREW) known as CETEC now act as a Coordination Unit for IRIS. The original purpose of the IRIS network is set out in Table 8.2.

Table 8.2.   IRIS: women's training network

Objectives of IRIS	
1	To increase the provision of good-quality training for women
2	To publicise women's training needs, promote exchanges of information and experience, develop cooperation and identify potential partners
3	To evaluate and develop training programmes adapted to the needs of women
4	To increase the involvement of employers and trade unions in vocational training programmes for women

Source: Commission of the European Communities (1991) *Equal Opportunities for Women and Men: Social Europe Supplement 3/91* Directorate General for Employment Industrial Relations and Social Affairs, Luxembourg: Office for Official Publications of the European Communities

The IRIS network encourages the exchange of methodologies and practices among those who train women. It provides an information service, undertakes some training activities itself, is consulted on issues regarding women's training by the EC and other organisations, runs summer schools, and publishes reports on key issues, such as the under-utilisation of women (Franceskides and de Troy 1994) and evaluation techniques (IRIS n.d.).[4]

The IRIS network Coordination Unit is a source of information on innovative training projects for women throughout the EU, and is strongly supported by the Advisory Committee on Equal Opportunities for Women and Men and the Women's Lobby in the European Parliament. The funding from the Commission for the IRIS network, which was never substantial (see Table 7.1), ceased in 1995 and was replaced by a system of subscriptions from members. This has reduced the number of members (to about 300) and makes the future of the network more susceptible to the fortunes of its members, many of whom operate in the precariously-funded third sector, and its ability to generate funding from other activities such as running LEONARDO DA VINCI projects. Its privatisation may be seen as a casualty of mainstreaming, where support for women's spaces is withdrawn on the grounds that positive action is no longer needed.

One of the observations which can be made from the projects in the IRIS network is how vital are what are known as 'supplementary measures' to the success of women's training. These include guidance and counselling, confidence-building, developing direct links with the labour market, improving knowledge of labour market information, training in job-seeking, childcare, family-friendly hours and so on. Numerous studies have witnessed the significance of these activities in assisting women, particularly women returners and those with disadvantages, to reintegrate into the labour market (Deroure 1990). Lefebvre (1993), too, draws attention to the need for 'accompanying measures', which are a characteristic of positive action projects for women, to become part of standard provision. She identifies both 'upstream' accompanying measures, such as EO training awareness for employers, and 'downstream' ones, such as guidance, access and childcare support for women. If these were integrated into training provision, women's participation might increase.

Overall, we can see that the approach to EO in the ESF is *laissez-faire*, with a model of equal treatment supplemented with some positive action. There is inadequate gender monitoring. Patterns of participation appear to reflect and reinforce those of gender segregation in the labour market. Positive action projects and the IRIS network have provided and disseminated examples of good practice. As yet, however, the extent to which the ESF is being used to develop women's training is limited. Some of these patterns are also characteristic of the EC's action programme on training, LEONARDO DA VINCI.

LEONARDO DA VINCI

LEONARDO DA VINCI, the EC's action programme on training, is aimed at developing the human resources of the EU's workforce. The programme is designed to run from 1995 to 2000 and there is an annual call for proposals published by the EC. The applications are managed by a Technical Assistance Office (TAO) based in Brussels and supported by a National Coordination Unit (NCU) in each Member State.

A key element of LEONARDO projects is that they should be transnational. Partners, who *inter alia* may include education and training providers, employers and trade unions, local authorities and regional bodies, work in partnerships to develop and disseminate information on innovative approaches to developing skills.

Projects should also be innovative. However, what has already been tested in one country or sector or context can still be regarded as 'innovative' if it is tried elsewhere, or in another sector, so the operationalisation of the concept of innovation is a permissive one. Harrison (1996) has argued, with regard to projects funded under the Community Initiatives, that there is no consensus in the EC as to what constitutes 'innovation'. This means that opportunities to learn from pilot projects may be lost.

Successful applications must also fall under one of the Commission's 'priority themes'. These are in part an echo of broad themes that characterised the previous generation of action programmes (described in Chapter 7) but also reflect the concerns of the Ruberti guidelines (CEC 1993f) and the *Teaching and Learning* White Paper (EC 1996b). They tend, so far at least, not to change much from year to year. Priority themes for 1996/7 are detailed in Table 8.3.

These themes include references to key concepts such as social exclusion and lifelong learning, which are fundamental to all three

Table 8.3.   Priority themes for LEONARDO DA VINCI 1996/97

1	Acquisition of new skills
2	Links between education and training establishments and enterprises
3	Combating exclusion
4	Promoting investment in human resources
5	Promoting access to skills through the information society in the context of lifelong learning

White Papers on economic, social, and teaching and learning policy (these White Papers and their underlying themes are discussed in the next chapter).

Administratively, LEONARDO is arranged under a number of 'strands', under which 'promoters' (transnational teams of project applicants) can make bids. These are set out in Table 8.4.

The chances of success for potential applicants is not very high. In response to the first call for proposals in 1995, some 4,540 applications were received, of which only 749 were funded (16.5 per cent). However, those funded were made up of partnerships of over 4,000 organisations. In 1996, there were 7,657 proposals, of which 1,542 were approved (14.6 per cent). These included 1,116 pilot projects, 291 placement and exchange projects, 47 multiplier projects and 88 surveys and analyses projects. Altogether 23,500 partners are involved in these co-funded activities across eighteen participating countries: the fifteen Member States plus Cyprus, Malta and Turkey (the countries waiting in the wings for membership) (figures supplied by the LEONARDO TAO).

It will be noticed that two of the sub-strands (I.1.d and II.1.d) are targeted at projects specifically aiming to address the issue of EO. Such 'spaces' did not exist in the action programmes outlined in the previous chapter, and they reflect a decision to include positive action within LEONARDO. DGXXII organises meetings for projects grouped under various clusters, and one on 'EO' projects was convened in 1996 (for 1995 projects). It became clear from the presentations made by projects, however, that the model of EO which informed them was either equal treatment or positive action. Only one of those which made a presentation could be described as a mainstreaming project, that is, one which was likely to have a lasting effect on systems and structures, as opposed simply to those who participated.

Table 8.4.   The strands of LEONARDO DA VINCI

Strand I	Support for the improvement of vocational training systems and arrangements in the Member States of the European Union and the countries of the European Economic Area (EEA)	

	I.1	Design and implementation of transnational pilot projects
		a) training of young people
		b) continuing vocational training
		c) vocational guidance
		d) equal opportunities for men and women
		e) training disadvantaged people
	I.2	Transnational placement and exchange programmes
		a) young trainees
		b) young workers
		c) trainers

Strand II	Support for the improvement of vocational training measures, including university/industry cooperation, concerning undertakings and workers	

	II.1	Transnational pilot projects
		a) innovation in training to take account of technological change
		b) investment in continuing training in companies
		c) university/industry cooperation in respect of transfer of technological innovation
		d) the promotion of equal opportunities for men and women in training
	II.2	Transnational placements and exchange programmes
		a) university students and new graduates
		b) personnel in companies and universities or training organisations
		c) people in charge of training

Strand III	Support for the development of language skills, knowledge and the dissemination of innovation in the field of vocational training	

	III.1	Development of language skills
		a) transnational pilot projects
		b) transnational exchanges
	III.2	Development of knowledge in the field of vocational training
		a) surveys and analyses
		b) exchange of comparable data
	III.3	Development of the dissemination of innovations in the field of vocational training
		a) multiplier-effect projects
		b) transnational exchange programmes

In addition to the sub-strands on EO, other initiatives have been taken in an attempt to promote EO within LEONARDO. At the briefing meetings for 1997 project applicants, held in Brussels in February 1997 and attended by over 500 promoters, workshops on how to mainstream EO were provided by DGXXII staff (and the author). All project promoters were reminded that they needed to be mindful of the EO dimension of their project. They were advised to formulate EO objectives for their project, identify means of monitoring progress, and specify methods of seeking to achieve their objectives. Promoters should then report on progress in this aspect of their work in their annual reports, and use EO as an internal evaluation criterion (see Guidelines to Promoters on EO in Appendix IV). The TAO will be using EO as a criterion in the external evaluation of projects.

To what extent this message will be heard over and above all the other messages on how to construct a successful application is hard to say. Nevertheless, building an expectation into the system of funding to which such a significant number of organisations throughout the EU look to resource projects may, at the very least, act as an awareness-raising exercise. However, it is clear from the nature of debates with project promoters at the EO cluster meeting, the 1997 Promoters Fair, and from the outputs of the previous action programmes featured in the Innovative Training Products Fair held in 1996 (EC 1996d, 1996e), that the potential for development of EO within LEONARDO, and the capacity for LEONARDO projects to influence practice within its organisations, is far from being fully exploited.

WOMEN-SPECIFIC PROJECTS

Numerous examples of EC co-funded good practice in women's training are available, from the IRIS network's 'models projects' to the EC and Social Partners *Compendium of Good Practice* (CEEP, ETUC and UNICE 1995). From these experiences, guides for promoters on running innovative and transnational projects have been drawn up (Blackley 1994; Blackley *et al.* 1995). This section gives an account of just three projects to illustrate the potential benefits of transnational work in the field of women's training.

The DIVA project is co-funded under LEONARDO and coordinated by the Welsh Development Agency. It builds upon a previous DGXXII-funded transnational FORCE project, ATHENA. In

ATHENA it was discovered that support agencies for people who wanted to set up their own businesses operated with a model of an entrepreneur that was exclusively male. Particular issues faced by women entrepreneurs were rarely or inadequately addressed. Research shows that these included a lack of experience and knowledge on financial management, lack of confidence, training needs, inability to raise start-up loans (partly because of lack of collateral), childcare needs while training or starting-up, and sometimes a desire to run a small business in such a way that childcare and other domestic responsibilities can be accommodated. If a woman wanted to run her business on a part-time basis, business support agencies rarely took her seriously (Rees 1992b: Chapter 8; Smith 1993a).

The DIVA project is working transnationally to produce a training video for business support agencies and finance houses which will alert them to the needs of women entrepreneurs and suggest imaginative ways of addressing these needs. It will be available in all the main Community languages and will include examples of good practice from different Member States. It invites business support agencies to look at their range of services from a gendered perspective. The long-term objective is to mainstream equal opportunities within these support agencies so that women entrepreneurs will be offered services which address their needs more exactly. Hence, the project seeks to achieve a long-term gain by changing the way in which services are delivered.

A second example is a LEONARDO DA VINCI surveys and analysis project on managing diversity called Project Mosaic.[5] Designed to learn from companies which maintain that they are actively engaged with managing diverse workforces, the idea is to document and analyse their practices with a view to an active dissemination phase and follow-up work, developing training materials for companies which want to follow their example. It falls into the LEONARDO priority theme of development of human resources.

The project is made up of three teams of partners from seven Member States. The core team comprise researchers from five Member States (UK, Sweden, Italy, Ireland, the Netherlands) who work together to develop the design of the project, conduct company case studies and analyse results. They will be collecting data from employers within their own Member States but will then draw upon the results of all the case studies to write thematic reports. The second tier of partners is made up of 'validators' from each of the original five countries and Greece, Germany, the Netherlands and Spain. They are made up of organisations such as equality agencies, personal development bodies, management institutes, regional authorities and trade union and employer bodies. Their function is to act as a sounding board for the core team, to assist in the identification of case study employers and to advise and help with dissemination and follow-up activities. The final team is made up of employers who already have a reputation for managing diverse workforces, and whose agreement to participate was necessary to demonstrate the feasibility for the project even though they will not all necessarily become case study companies. They will all, however, be involved in discussions of the results. The project, funded in the 1996 round, is seeking at a transnational level to develop expertise on mainstreaming equality, and indeed to go beyond gender to include other equality dimensions.

In the Structural Funds, the NOW strand of EMPLOYMENT is a reserved space for activities focused on women (see Callender 1994). This gave rise to a project on contract cleaning, principally involving Ireland and Denmark (see McAdam 1994); here I summarise the Irish part of the project. In 1991, a group of major employers in the Irish contract cleaning industry, together with a leading trade union, jointly undertook a pilot training and development programme centred on the needs of women in the industry under the NOW programme. About 150 women from six participating cleaning companies were involved; they were drawn from managerial, supervisory, union representative and cleaner levels in each organisation. Most worked part-time. McAdam reports that the contract cleaning industry employs 30,000 workers in Ireland in about 100 companies, varying in size from 10 to over 2,000 employees, and that the industry was identified as having growth potential.

The women worked together in identifying their skill needs and the skills they had that were not being used in work. This led to the expansion of services the employer was able to offer to customers, and to training leading to the enhancement of quality. As a consequence of this project and its innovative approach to learning and participation, it is maintained, a low-paid, female-dominated sector was able to improve quality and offer new services (McAdam 1994).

Within the ESF, then, and within LEONARDO, there are opportunities to move beyond equal treatment and positive action to seek to mainstream equal EO. Pressure to do so is coming directly from the Commission and is being supported by the Council of Ministers, as the following section shows. This could have a profound effect in the future upon both the ESF and LEONARDO.

MAINSTREAMING

There have been various signs in the changing discourse of the EC and European Parliament which indicate a shift in the underlying model of EO from one of equal treatment and then positive action towards mainstreaming. The most significant of these indications was the publication by the EC (1996) of a Communication to the Council of Ministers calling for the integration of EO into all Community actions, policies and programmes. This affects not simply ESF and LEONARDO but all the Structural Funds, and indeed all Community activities, internal and external. The implications of this Communication, which is designed to go much further than employment and training measures, are discussed in more detail in the final chapter.

The reform of the Structural Funds in 1993 was significant for the development of EO, in that a new standard regulation was introduced specifically referring to EO. Article 7 of the new regulation stated:

actions funded by the Structural Funds . . . or any other existing financial mechanism must conform to the content of the treaties and acts and rulings relating to them, as well as Community policies, including those relating to rules governing competition, the according of public contracts and the protection of the environment, along with the respect of the principle of equal opportunities between women and men.

(cited in EC 1997: 22)

The principle of EO features in all the documentation for the Community Initiatives such as EMPLOYMENT, ADAPT and ADAPT-BIS.

The rules governing the Structural Funds have obliged all concerned to take EO into account since 1993, but the Communication adds further force to this. The Commissioner with special responsibility for the ERDF, Monika Wulf-Matheis, has refused to fund bids from Member States in the last year that were gender-neutral or did not take sufficiently seriously the equality dimension. Hence the Communication is beginning to have some impact. As she has said with reference to Objective 2 programmes, EO is one of the Commission's four priorities, and she 'will make sure that no programme is approved which does not include measures promoting equal opportunities' (Wulf-Matheis 1997: 7).

Tracing the history of this through the various Presidencies, some key steps can be identified. The outgoing Greek Presidency in 1994 put forward a Resolution to the EU Social Affairs Ministers which calls on Member States to *ensure* (my emphasis) that EO for women and men are actively promoted in Structural Fund initiatives, especially those pursued under the ESF. The resolution, which includes references to targets for women and mainstreaming EO, was adopted. The Essen summit in 1995 decided that the promotion of EO was one of the fundamental tasks of the EU. Hence the ESF is now described as having to 'promote' EO as one of its specific objectives (Jones 1996) as opposed simply to offering equal treatment to men and women. The mainstreaming message was further reinforced at a seminar on 'Structural Funds and Equal Opportunities' jointly organised by the EC and the Belgian government during the Belgian Presidency in Brussels in March 1996, and again at a follow-up conference during the Irish Presidency held in Dublin later that year.

The Dublin conference focused on the sharing of good practice, and encouraged the participation of people involved in EO in monitoring committees and evaluation procedures at the national level. The Irish Presidency has also proposed a Resolution on Equal Opportunities and Structural Funds which is expected to be adopted shortly. Hence, the mainstreaming agenda has been moved forward through a succession of Presidencies. It remains to be seen whether this trend will be followed or bucked by the upcoming UK Presidency in the first half of 1998. The attention to mainstreaming through the various Member State Presidencies has been reflected in the European Parliament. For example, the Women's Rights Committee organised a hearing on mainstreaming and the Structural Funds in 1996.

The Commissioner responsible for Employment and Social Affairs, Padraig Flynn, emphasised the need for positive action measures to continue alongside the mainstreaming process during his speech to the Dublin event (Flynn 1996). However, in the same speech, he announced the 'streamlining' of the nine equality networks (described in Chapter 4) down to two: one looking at legal issues, and the other on gender and employment. These are to be supplemented by groups of experts called together to examine specific themes (Flynn 1996: 5). Many have viewed this streamlining with some concern: the danger that mainstreaming will be used as a reason to discontinue positive action measures is ever present.

This fresh emphasis on EO in the Structural Funds, and an increased focus on synergy between the Funds, create new opportunities for projects which can incorporate some of the 'supplementary measures' outlined by Lefebvre (1993). For example, while ESF can be used to pay for the operating costs of education and training activity, the ERDF can be accessed for purchasing equipment and plant, for example for childcare facilities, afterschool care, and transport: all extremely important to enable women to take up training opportunities.

The enhanced emphasis on evaluation, with EO as a criteria, and the building of EO interests into monitoring committees and programme documents, should help to put EO on the agenda for Member States' multi-annual employment programmes. Some of these developments echo measures being taken in LEONARDO DA VINCI following the mainstreaming communication.

CONCLUSION

There are indications of a shift in thinking about EO in the design and implementation of both the ESF and LEONARDO. The extent to which this filters through to influence practice in projects is, of course, open to question. Moreover, the principle of subsidiarity and the desire to respect the 'rich diversity' of culture within the EU necessarily impact upon how projects approach the issue of EO. In Greece and Denmark, for example, positive action projects are thin on the ground. In the case of Greece, this is because the climate is not yet right for the widescale introduction of such measures; in Denmark, the low application for NOW projects is because the thinking there has moved beyond positive action. It is also the case that, while the mainstreaming agenda may be influencing some applications for Structural Funds, in particular ERDF where Commissioner Wulf-Matheis is particularly keen to see mainstreaming introduced, this enthusiasm is far from necessarily being shared by key actors and gatekeepers in the localities, regions and Member States – or, of course, in all quarters of the NCUs, the TAOs and Commission itself.

The mainstreaming agenda also has to be balanced as a priority against others that have emerged from the recent White Papers. How is the focus on EO for men and women matched against the political priority of combating social exclusion – a concept that appears to focus on meeting the needs of identified disadvantaged groups? And how does combating exclusion square with enhancing economic competitiveness and developing human resources? These questions are the focus of the next chapter.

Chapter 9

Competitiveness, social exclusion and the learning society
EO and the White Papers[1]

While perusing the instructions at a U-Bahn ticket machine at Bonn station one cold Sunday night last February, I was surrounded by what I took to be a small group of dishevelled elderly men seeking to assist me in working out the fare to my destination. On closer inspection, and having noticed ragged sleeping bags and blankets in evidence, it became clear that the men were in fact of diverse ages but had aged prematurely as a consequence of some time spent sleeping rough. Moreover, it became evident that, although they were more than willing to attempt to offer interpretations of the instructions on the ticket machine, their prime purpose in approaching me was to solicit small change. Having dispensed some limited largesse, I settled down, alone on the platform, to wait the half hour before the train was due.

While waiting, I read my copy of *The Big Issue Cymru* [Wales] magazine, purchased some hours earlier at Cardiff station from a cheerful young man, also inadequately protected from the cold, and also homeless. *The Big Issue Cymru* (and its sister publications in Scotland and some regions of England) was set up to provide an opportunity for homeless people to make an income; by becoming official vendors, they can keep the difference between what they pay for copies of the magazine and its sale price to the public. *The Big Issue Cymru* also gives a voice to homeless people in its pages, providing insight into their lives through letters, articles and poems. It features in each edition old photographs of four people who are 'missing', asking them to get in touch with family and friends. They all tell a story of someone whose contact with both kith and kin and with mainstream organisations, institutions and agencies appears to have become highly tenuous and then been severed altogether.

The lives of the 'missing' which appeared in *The Big Issue Cymru* put me in mind of the study by researchers at the University of Wales, Cardiff, mentioned in Chapter 5 (Istance *et al.* 1994; Rees *et al.* 1996). They were commissioned by South Glamorgan Training and Enterprise Council to estimate how many 16 to 18-year-olds were not in education, training or employment, and to find out what they were doing. Young people in this age group have not been eligible for unemployment benefit since a change in the regulations in the UK in 1988. It is intended that they stay on in education, move into employment, take up a training course or accept a place on the Government's Youth Training Scheme. The research project was inevitably problematic; by definition, counting and describing the activities of a group of people who do not appear on any lists demanded the imaginative use and interpretation of a surrogate indicator – in this case, secondary analysis of careers service records. Nevertheless, the calculations were made and some qualitative research was conducted with young people identified as not being in education, training or employment.

A small number of those successfully traced were interviewed and found to be 'making out', to a greater or lesser extent, through a series of activities. Some had turned to the hidden economy or to crime, a few of whom were earning more than they would be likely to receive on Youth Training and possibly developing a wider range of skills, albeit ones whose transferability to legitimate employment might be somewhat limited. A few were in prison or on remand. Some were into drugs. Some young women had become teenage mothers and were as a consequence able to access subsistence level support from the state. Others were homeless, dossing on friends' floors, begging on the street and so on. As other research in South Wales has shown, many young homeless people have been 'in care' and therefore have no families to which to return (Hutson and Liddiard 1994). Most of the young people whose existence was indicated in the statistical analysis of the careers service records were, of course, untraceable. Some may have left the area or, indeed, died.

One of the most shocking aspects of this study, however, was that the researchers calculated that, at any one time, up to a fifth of young people in this age group could be described as having 'disappeared'. In other words, they were not in contact with the range of state agencies which exist to assist people in the transition from education to working life. Just under half of the 'disappeared' were young women (Istance *et al.* 1994). This is eerily redolent of biographies of some (although by no means all) of the victims of the Wests, the Gloucestershire mass murderers, young women not engaged with organisations and institutions, and not readily recognised as missing.

The interaction between patterns of industrial restructuring in the South Wales labour market, which has reduced the demand for youth labour, and changes in the welfare system, which removed the right of these young people to unemployment benefit, has resulted in a sizeable group of 16 to 18-year-olds moving beyond the reach of statutory and voluntary agencies. Moreover, there is no particular reason to think that this part of South Wales is different from other parts of the UK or indeed the rest of Europe in this regard (Wilkinson 1995). The size and nature of the phenomenon of the young 'disappeared' is an issue about which we know very little.

The intensification of competitive pressures and the impact of the global economy have led to complex patterns of industrial restructuring, and have produced an increasingly varied and fast-changing set of occupational lifechances for those entering the labour market and those leaving it prematurely, as well as for employees and the unemployed. The state of the economy and the interaction between economic and social welfare policies can exacerbate or ameliorate the chances of individuals, groups, localities and regions of becoming separated from the rest of society in terms of standard of living and involvement in activities and institutions. While for some, individual incomes soar to unprecedented levels (the earnings and bonuses of those in the privatised utilities in the UK provide examples here), for others it is clear that welfare systems designed in the early post-war period to provide a short-term safety net for crisis situations are inadequate for the task of sustaining considerable numbers of people for an indefinite period. While the unemployment register has always consisted of different people moving in and out of a pool, there is now an increasing number of long-term unemployed for whom joblessness and subsistence living is a way of life for the foreseeable future. Moreover, an increasing number of people at either end of the working age-range are squeezed out of the labour market through a combination of changes in the welfare system and refocusing of labour demand. Growing polarisation between job-rich and job-poor constitutes the crisis challenging the Single European Market. Young people, women and middle-aged/older men are particularly at risk of unemployment.

The term now in common currency in the EC to describe what these jobless individuals are experiencing is 'social exclusion'. And indeed not just individuals, but households, localities and whole regions, are deemed at risk. But what is social exclusion? And is its avoidance compatible with achieving a competitive economy? How does social exclusion differ from old fashioned poverty or multiple deprivation? And how do policies designed to reduce or eradicate social exclusion relate to those intended to ensure that men and women are treated equally?

This chapter seeks to address these questions. It begins by discussing the shift in the conceptualisation of 'social exclusion'. It then gives an account of the approach of the EU to developing strategies for the future through its three White Papers which set the framework for the development of policy for the foreseeable future. The first is on economic policy, which focuses on developing economic competitiveness and reducing unemployment (EC 1994a). The second is on social policy, which concentrates on the avoidance of social exclusion among citizens of the EU (EC 1994b). The third is on developing a 'learning society' through education, training and skill development (EC 1996b). The chapter concludes with some observations on the relationship between social exclusion and EO policies.

THE CONCEPT OF SOCIAL EXCLUSION

In the 1960s and 1970s, those left without work as a result of patterns of industrial restructuring, whether individuals, families or regions, were among those described as being 'poor'. Poverty in the UK was dramatically rediscovered among the general affluence of post-war society in the 1960s (Townsend 1979). State action programmes were launched to combat poverty, both in European countries and the US. In the UK in the late 1970s, locally-based action research Community Development Projects were funded by the Home Office, intended to assist people in such 'deprived' communities to get back on their feet.[2] The EC funded three of its own Anti-Poverty Programmes, in the mid-1970s, the late 1980s and the early 1990s (Room 1995). However, analyses of all these various programmes pointed beyond the need to help the 'poor' to the recognition that multiple deprivation was the result of tensions between shifts in capital and the shaping of the welfare state. Poverty was thus recognised as being multi-dimensional and an outcome of external pressures, rather than the result of the personal inadequacies of those who found themselves in straitened circumstances.

This reinforcement of divisions between rich and poor individuals, households, localities and regions is one of the major consequences of industrial change and the intensification of competitive pressures. Competitions inevitably produce winners and losers, as Weber (1968) observed:

> Usually one group of competitors takes some externally identifiable characteristic of another group of (actual or potential) competitors – race, language, religion, local or social origin, descent, resident etc – as a pretext for attempting their exclusion. It does not matter which characteristic is chosen in the individual case: whatever suggests itself most easily is seized upon.
>
> (Weber 1968: 242, cited in Brown and Crompton 1994: 5)

The 'insiders' form an interest group against the outsiders. Brown and Crompton (1994) argue that there are two types of 'outsiders': the first is where the rules of exclusion are based upon group membership, while the second is individual-based. In the EU, the most obvious group of 'outsiders' are non-citizens: that is, refugees, migrants and guestworkers and their families who are resident but are not afforded citizen status and the rights that pertain to that status (see Chapter 5).

Other residents who do enjoy citizen status may nevertheless become excluded in that they are denied full participation in social, cultural and economic life, on either a group or an individual basis. Groups are defined by membership of a class, gender or race, or by sexual orientation, language, disability or other defining factor. The effects of exclusion may be manifested in lack of access to resources, but the concept of social exclusion is wider than the notion of poverty. It is also broader than the idea of multiple deprivation, which incorporates the 'housing poor', the 'transport poor' and the 'access poor' and their combinations with the more traditional understanding of absolute poverty as being simply without sufficient resource to sustain life.

The notion of social exclusion, then, appears to incorporate the lack of opportunity to participate in the structures and institutions of society. Room (1995: 6) detects a conceptual difference between what he describes as the Anglo-Saxon notion of poverty and the French tradition of social analysis which is the basis for the concept of social exclusion. The concept of poverty, he argues, is associated with the liberal philosophical tradition and rooted in a distributional notion, where individuals must be equipped with sufficient resources to compete in the market place. By contrast, the vision of social exclusion propounded by the French (or more broadly by the intellectuals and political elites of continental Europe), he says, is one where society is seen as:

> a status hierarchy or as a number of collectivities, bound together by sets of mutual rights and obligations that are rooted in some broader moral order.

> (Room 1995: 6)

Social exclusion, according to Room, is the process of becoming detached from this moral order.

The agenda for social analysis, then, is to examine how systems which contribute to the way in which individuals acquire their cultural and human capital, skills and qualifications disadvantage or advantage people with particular sets of ascriptive characteristics. To what extent do such systems reproduce advantage for some groups and disadvantage for others? And to what extent do social, economic, and education and training policies address and indeed redress these tendencies? It is with this question in mind that the focus now turns to the three recent EC White Papers.

THE WHITE PAPERS

The issue of social exclusion is high on the agenda of the EU. Berghman (1995: 11) has traced the etymology of the term from its first appearance in an EC document published towards the end of the second European poverty programme in 1988 to its inclusion in the European Social Charter, in the Maastricht Treaty, as an objective of the Structural Funds, as part of the Fourth Framework Research Programme and as integral to LEONARDO DA VINCI and SOCRATES, the training and education action programmes of the EC. Indeed, one of the many European Observatories the EC has established is on Policies to Combat Social Exclusion (see Robbins *et al.* 1994).

In the mid-1990s, the three White Papers were produced, designed respectively to enhance competitiveness, reduce unemployment and combat social exclusion, and to foster a skilled workforce in a knowledge-based society (EC 1994a; 1994b; 1996b). They outline the shape of social, economic, and education and training policies for the EU in the 1990s. The Delors White Paper on economic policy, *Growth, Competitiveness, Employment: The Challenges and Ways Forward into the 21st Century* (EC 1994a), named after Frenchman Jacques Delors, a previous President of the EU, focuses on the development of economic competitiveness and the avoidance of unemployment in the context of the Single Market. The 'Flynn' White Paper on social policy, *European Social Policy: A Way Forward for the Union* (EC 1994b), named after Irishman Padraig Flynn, Commissioner for Employment and Social Affairs, concentrates on the avoidance of 'social exclusion'. The 'Cresson' White Paper on *Teaching and Learning: Towards The Learning Society* (EC 1996b), named after Frenchwoman Edith Cresson, Commissioner for Research, Education and Training, sets out an agenda to turn the EU into a learning society.

The essence of the White Papers is that, to prosper and, indeed, to survive, the EU must develop a highly trained and flexible workforce where the potential of human resources is developed to the full. In this way, economic competitiveness can be enhanced, unemployment reduced and a decent standard of living achieved for all citizens. It is of paramount importance, all the Papers emphasise, to reduce unemployment significantly, and with it social exclusion.

However, Levitas (1996) argues that the concept of social exclusion as discussed in the (first two) EC White Papers – and, indeed, in the report of the Commission on Social Justice in the UK (Commission on Social Justice 1994) – is too narrowly focused. By defining social exclusion entirely in terms of the labour market, the significance of other aspects of social life, such as unpaid work, is diminished. Moreover, the bifurcation into 'included' and 'excluded' suggests a homogeneity of the included which the evidence suggests is unwarranted. Hence, inequalities among those in employment are obscured by a focus on the relationship between the employed and the unemployed. By the same token, the focus on social exclusion and its corollaries, social integration and cohesion, by definition also diminishes the amount of attention paid to those outside the labour market, such as children, people with full-time unpaid caring and domestic responsibilities, the retired and the chronically sick. The pursuit of social integration defined exclusively in terms of the labour market, Levitas argues, thus draws attention away from other forms of social inequality.

It is true to say that all three White Papers focus to a greater or lesser extent on the labour market, and that social exclusion is largely defined in those terms. Hence, education and training are identified as the key to the future – to the enhanced competitiveness of the Single Market, to the avoidance of social exclusion, and to the development of a knowledge-based society. But the forms of inequality which characterise both education and training systems and the labour market, and which are arguably endemic in capitalist economies, are ignored in the White Paper.

The particular dimension of inequality upon which I wish to focus is the most obvious one, that of gender. Despite the significance of gender as a key determinant in who receives what education and training, in what subject and with what implication for future employment prospects, all three White Papers on the surface appear to be almost entirely gender-neutral.

As Levitas (1996) remarks, the definition of social exclusion in terms simply of unemployment obscures poverty among women who are economically inactive and in old age. On average they earn less than men during their working lives and have a longer period of life expectancy in old age. Poverty among elderly women has been linked in a number of studies to pension schemes designed for men working continuously and full-time (Arber and Ginn 1991; Ginn and Arber 1996), and to women having to live for more years on state rather than occupational pensions (Wenger 1995). As women tend to be responsible for the major share of unpaid work in the family, this constrains their ability to sell their labour in the market place. Women also comprise the majority (84 per cent) of single parents (Eurostat 1992). Cumulatively, then, women constitute the majority of the poor.

A focus on inequality between those in and out of employment also obscures inequalities between those in work. Gender segregation in the labour force is one of its most highly sustained characteristics, and yet the policies do not seek to address this issue. As we have seen, women have higher unemployment rates and are the majority of the economically inactive, new labour market entrants, and those engaged in 'atypical work', such as part-time contracts, low-paid work and temporary employment (Meulders *et al.* 1994). Equal treatment policies have failed to make much impact on the rigidity of these patterns.

GROWTH, COMPETITIVENESS, EMPLOYMENT

The economic White Paper, *Growth, Competitiveness, Employment*, is by far the longest of the three. It was the first to be published and it presents a detailed analysis of the changing labour market structures of the EU and identifies as a major priority the need to generate jobs to combat unemployment (EC 1994a). The paper was discussed by the Council of Ministers at the Brussels summit (concluding the Belgian Presidency) in December 1993, at which time seven themes were identified as the main focus for follow up activities: improving education and training systems; improving flexibility within companies and in the labour market; developing formulas for the reorganisation of work; reducing indirect costs of labour, particularly for unskilled work; making better use of public funds for combating unemployment; developing special measures for young untrained people; and developing new jobs on the basis of new needs. These themes were the subject of debates at the Essen Summit of the German Presidency in December 1994, and they have formed the focus of further follow-up activities.

The document expresses a commitment to equal treatment of men and women but is otherwise largely silent on the issue of gender. No doubt in response to this, the Equal Opportunities Unit in DGV commissioned seven academics (known as the 'seven wise women') from across the EU to provide, in preparation for the Essen Summit in 1994, a feminist critique of plans outlined in the White Paper (EC 1995d; Rees 1995a).[3] We were each asked to concentrate on one of seven themes broadly comparable to those listed above: education and training (Rees 1995a); inequalities and flexibilities (Maruani 1995); reorganisation of work (Meulders 1995); gender, employment and working time (Beccalli and Salvati 1995); wage and non-wage labour costs, social security and public funds to combat unemployment (Maier 1995); youth unemployment and the condition of young women in the labour market (Pugliese 1995); and EO and requirements for new jobs (de Bruijn 1995).

The ensuing critique demonstrated the androcentricity of the thinking behind the White Paper and revealed many of the limitations of a gender-neutral approach to an economy where gender plays such a significant role (EC 1995c). To be effective, as de Bruijn (1995: 111) concluded, equality policies need to be integrated into labour market analysis and policies, rather than tacked on:

it means more than making references to women's employment and to equal opportunities. It also means more than just paying special attention to women as a target group as the White Paper does. Analysing from a gender perspective implies that on the one hand gender inequalities should be examined as one of the causes of developments in employment and unemployment. On the other hand gender inequalities could also be produced by 'general' labour market developments and policies. The White Paper does pay some attention to the first, but not to the latter.

The analysis of labour market change in the White Paper ignores its gendered aspects. For example, the point is made that, when new jobs are created, it is new labour force entrants that seem to take them rather than the registered unemployed: creating new jobs, therefore, does not always reduce unemployment. A gendered analysis would show that the majority of these new workers are women who are the 'hidden unemployed'. Second, while the Paper describes sectoral changes, it does not draw attention to the fact that, in the loss of manufacturing jobs and the gain of service sector jobs, not only does this represent a shift towards women's employment, but it also means a deterioration of work contracts among the employed. Women are not simply segregated from men in terms of the occupations and sectors within which they work, but also in the hours and type of contracts they have. Hence, sectoral shifts, and the gender changes in the workforce these have produced, have led to an overall deterioration in pay levels and terms and conditions of those in employment. Finally, while concern is expressed at the loss of low-skilled jobs due to the shift in demand towards a more skill-based workforce, it is in fact largely male low-skilled work that has disappeared. Other low-paid (deemed low-skilled) work that has been the reserve of women has not declined, indeed it has increased. But only those for whom such work and its meagre remuneration can constitute a secondary income can afford to work in such jobs. This tends to restrict such opportunities to young people, who expect to move on, or women whose income is supplemented by a man or by the state. Hence, a policy devoted to increasing low-paid jobs will not, in fact, affect the problem of male unemployment.

This financial dependence of women either on men or on welfare benefits, on which employers paying low wages depend, underlies a fundamental point made in a recent OECD (1994) report on women and the labour market. It concluded that new employment and gender contracts need to be constructed to replace that of the male breadwinner/female homemaker which underlies much current labour market, care and welfare policy. Hence, without paying attention to welfare, taxation and the care economy, and without addressing the gender imbalance between responsibility for domestic work and caring, altering labour market polices alone will not resolve the problem of balancing home and work faced by women. It will not allow women to participate in the labour market in the way in which both the White Paper and the OECD suggest is required for a competitive economy.

The contributors to the feminist critique of the White Paper also pointed out other examples of androcentric thinking. They argued, for example, that the concern expressed about unemployment is implicitly concern about male unemployment. Similarly, the White Paper's advocacy of reducing non-wage employment costs in order to create jobs assumes a male starting point, from which there is some scope to level down. However, millions of women already work in unprotected, part-time, low-paid work.

The three main proposals for a long-term strategy for equality in the labour market which emerge from this document are: the necessity for complementary policies to address the balance between home and work (for example, caring, taxation and welfare); the advisability in terms of EO to opt for a reduced full working week rather than a combination of 'super-full-time' workers and a flexible workforce; and, finally, instituting minimum wages and wage bargaining procedures in more Member States, as they appear to be effective in reducing gender segregation in low-paid jobs.

The White Paper is essentially about economic growth, while seeking to maintain a commitment to equal treatment of men and women. Unfortunately, because the analysis is uninformed by gender, so too are the policies. As a consequence, the former cannot be achieved without the sacrifice of the latter.

EUROPEAN SOCIAL POLICY

The second White Paper, *European Social Policy: A Way Forward for the Union* (EC 1994b), builds on the foundation laid in the economic White Paper and in responses (EC 1994e) to the earlier Green Paper, *European Social Policy: Options for the Future* (CEC 1993e). It identifies its guiding themes as partnership, subsidiarity and the redistribution of income and opportunities. The main emphasis is on a shift away from the management of unemployment towards the promotion of job creation and broadening access to work. Rather than increasing the income of those in work, the focus, it argues, should be on creating new jobs and bringing excluded groups into employment. While some might argue with this interpretation, the view expressed in the document is that the intention is not to dilute the European model of social protection, but to adapt, rationalise and simplify regulations, and to establish a better balance between social protection, competitiveness and employment creation.

This document recognises the complex nature of exclusion and says far more about EO than either of the other two White Papers. A Eurostat calculation suggests that there are 52 million people living below the poverty line in the EU.[4] This is attributed in the White Paper to structural change and is described as threatening the social cohesion of each Member State and the EU as a whole (EC 1994b: 49). The multi-faceted nature of social exclusion is acknowledged thus:

> Exclusion processes are dynamic and multidimensional in nature. They are linked not only to unemployment and/or to low incomes, but also to housing conditions, levels of education and opportunities, health, discrimination, citizenship and integration into the local community. As a result, preventing and combating social exclusion calls for an overall mobilization of effort and combination of both economic and social measures. At the European level, this also implies that social exclusion should be addressed in the framework of all Union policies.

In response to this situation, and because of the need to draw the excluded 'in' and prevent others from becoming excluded, two new Community Initiatives were introduced into the ESF to promote adaptation to industrial change. The EMPLOYMENT Community Initiative is aimed at special target groups among the socially excluded: young people (YOUTHSTART), women (NOW), and the disabled (HORIZON). ADAPT (and now, ADAPT-BIS), aimed at workers at risk of unemployment because of industrial change (these were both discussed in Chapter 8). These Community Initiatives, however, account for a very small proportion of the Structural Funds overall, and even of the ESF.

The White Paper does have a gender dimension, indeed a whole chapter is devoted to EO between men and women. However, this again means that EO is seen as a separate, rather than an integrated, dimension of policy. EO is identified as one of the five 'shared values' of the European social model, along with democracy and individual rights, free collective bargaining, a market economy and social welfare and solidarity (EC 1994b: 9). The significance of EO is emphasised in terms not simply of social justice but of the need to maximise use made of human resources for a competitive economy, in view of the increase in female economic activity rates and the changing family structure. Moreover, the text includes a recognition of the limited effect of EO approaches so far:

> Experience now shows that formal equal opportunities alone do not automatically result in either equal treatment or proper representation of women at decision-making levels. Closer examination is required of the entrenched institutional and cultural barriers that inhibit or prevent the proportional representation of women in public and political bodies including organization of the social partners. The European Union should exercise leadership by taking concrete steps to enhance the role of women in its own institutions and should assist the Member States and the other European institutions to make progress in the same direction.
>
> (EC 1994b: 43,44)

The White Paper also acknowledges that there are differences among women and that there is an urgent need to desegregate the labour market. The necessity of integrating specific social objectives into the strategic plans of business are mentioned in this regard. The potential role the Social Partners can fulfil through, for example, costing positive action and family-friendly measures and providing practical guidelines is underlined. The document identifies stereotyping, gender monitoring, gender-neutral job evaluation and job classification schemes and the need to move more women into decision-making positions as areas that the EC needs to address. The merits of positive action are acknowledged and the significance of cultural barriers recognised, but the steps advocated towards combating discrimination and pursuing EO remain largely rooted in the liberal tradition of equal treatment.

The social policy White Paper breaks new ground in that it begins to address wider dimensions of EO by referring to race, religion, age and disability. It makes clear that the Commission has no competence on these issues but that 'serious consideration must be given to the introduction of a specific reference to combating discrimination on the grounds of race, religion, age and disability' at the next opportunity to revise the Treaties (EC 1994b: 52).

The Paper is informed, therefore, by gender, in that the fact that women are the majority of those experiencing exclusion is acknowledged, although the extent to which this is in effect group exclusion is not. A main aim expressed in the policies presented is the need to desegregate the labour market; however, this is not accompanied by an analysis of how patterns of segregation are perpetuated or, therefore, by proposals which would be likely to have an effect upon them. It acknowledges that there are other dimensions to discrimination in the labour market and points to the need to address the Commission's limited competence in this regard in the next revision of the Treaties, but falls short of pointing to the concerns of those who responded to the Green Paper on Social Policy (CEC 1993b; EC 1994e; CREW n.d.).

TEACHING AND LEARNING POLICY

The White Paper on *Teaching and Learning: Towards the Learning Society* (EC 1996b) identifies three factors of 'upheaval' that need to be addressed through education and training: the impact of the information society; internationalisation; and a 'scientific and technical world' (EC 1995a: 5,6). All these factors, it is argued, make a strong case for serious commitment to learning, and indeed for a cultural change to valuing vocational training as much as education. A broad-based education for all is seen as essential for enhancing the employability of the EU's citizens, followed by systems and attitudes that can deliver lifelong learning.

Five objectives are set out: encouraging the acquisition of new knowledge; bringing schools and the business sector closer together; combating exclusion; proficiency in three languages; and treating material investment and investment in training on an equal basis. The White Paper clarifies what are seen as appropriate roles for the Commission and the Member States in the light of the principle of subsidiarity, and describes its overall objective as being 'in conjunction with the education and training policies of the Member States, to help Europe move towards the knowledge-based society' (EC 1996b: 11).

There is considerable emphasis in the White Paper on the need for flexibility on behalf of individuals, who need to develop a more positive attitude to learning after the end of their full-time compulsory education. Similarly, more adaptability is required on the part of education and training providers, the social partners, regional and national authorities and funding bodies, to create a more open set of opportunities for individuals to pursue learning. In effect the Paper is arguing that new routes of progression need to be built between institutions which traditionally have offered separate trajectories.

Specific proposals are made for each of the five objectives. To encourage the acquisition of new knowledge, European networks of research centres, vocational training providers and companies will be set up to identify the skills and knowledge areas that need to be provided for future needs. In addition, 'personal skill cards' will be developed to provide individuals with a permanent record of their knowledge and levels and areas of skill which can be updated to show to prospective employers. In order to develop closer links between schools and the business sector, apprenticeships will be developed and apprenticeship centres in the various Member States will be networked to provide opportunities for exchanges among apprentices, similar to those available to students under the ERASMUS programme. An apprentices' charter will be introduced to aid mobility. To combat exclusion, second-chance community-based schools will be provided in 'problem' areas, targeted at those for whom school did not prove an effective place to learn, and funded by monies redeployed from LEONARDO DA VINCI and SOCRATES. To deliver the objective of improving the proficiency of EU citizens in three Community languages, a 'School of Europe' quality label is proposed for those schools which have proved to be successful in teaching languages to young people. Such schools will be networked. Finally, in support of the aim to treat material investment and investment in training on an equal basis, firms who invest in training will be encouraged in this activity by having this acknowledged in their balance sheets as an intangible asset. 'Training funds' will be developed for individuals wishing to increase their knowledge and skills.

Adult guidance acts as a broker between the individual and the education, training and labour market opportunities on offer and clearly has an increasingly important role to play in the context of an ageing workforce, a complex and fast-changing labour market and the Single Market. The significance of guidance is identified in the White Paper, where it is maintained that, at the moment, the 'citizen of Europe has better information when choosing a hotel or restaurant than when choosing a type of training.' (EC 1996b: 34). Some measures have already been introduced to develop adult guidance and counselling at the European level and to develop links between existing guidance services in the Member States.

The White Paper on Teaching and Learning, like the other two, acknowledges the principle of equal treatment of men and women as an objective. However, again, the policies presented are not particularly informed by the gendered nature of education, training provision or guidance services. EO is expressed as an idea and an ideal. More concrete proposals are made for tackling groups identified as socially disadvantaged. Unfortunately, the force of commitment to EO for men and women expressed in the document with some frequency is rather undermined by the use (in the English language version at least) of sexist language.

Education is identified as having played a key role in the 'emancipation' of women (p.16) and it is clearly true that the compulsory education of girls alongside that of boys has made a significant difference to women's participation in public life. The White Paper suggests that it is important to evaluate how 'training reduces segregation in the labour market by encouraging more women to enter traditionally male-dominated occupations' (p.35). While this would be a useful exercise, of course, training systems more generally perpetuate and indeed reinforce patterns of gender segregation in the labour market in ways described elsewhere in this book (and see Cockburn 1987). Courses designed to encourage women in non-traditional skills remain the exception rather than the rule, and are more likely to be found in short-term, precariously funded projects than in mainstream training provision.

There are other references to EO and to women in the document. For instance, it is recognised (p.36) that it is full-time employees of larger companies, and in particular senior managers and those employed in technological occupations and professions, who are most likely to be offered employer-sponsored training and that these are for the most part men.

The model of EO which underlies this White Paper appears to be the equal treatment model, with some recognition of the need for positive action and even positive discrimination in the case of non-traditional skills and, more particularly, to integrate the 'social disadvantaged'. It is clear that the major concern is about young people, especially in deprived urban areas which are identified as a target for special aid. Their 'integration' into the mainstream is identified as a priority. While the needs of such young men and women clearly are of concern, there is a missed opportunity to focus more explicitly on the training needs of women of all ages. For example, while one of the novel proposals presented in the White Paper is for 'second chance schools' for young people, this model could have been adopted for women who return to the labour market after a childbearing and rearing break. The tendency is for projects tailor-made for such women's needs to remain outside mainstream training provision, to be located in the third sector, and to be supported on an *ad hoc* basis by a series of grants from a variety of sources, including NOW and the ESF. South Glamorgan Women's Workshop in Cardiff, which targets disadvantaged women for training in technological and computing skills, is recognised as a model project by the EC-funded IRIS network of women's training projects, and has a list of distinguished visitors that reads like a European 'Who's Who' in training and EO, recently celebrated over ten years of existence: it nevertheless still has to complete grant application forms every year for the work it does and there is no guarantee that all or any of the funding bodies concerned will necessarily continue to support it.

Positive action, which has been an important part of the EC strategy for EO so far, is seen in the White Paper as an important mechanism for equal access for both men and women, but, even more so, for tackling social disadvantage more generally. Here, those living in rural communities, the elderly, ethnic minorities and immigrants are all mentioned specifically in the context of needing to ensure that they do not 'become second-class citizens as regards access to the new technologies and opportunities for learning' (EC 1996b: 37).

The White Paper clearly recognises inequalities in access to training and the labour market, and looks for possibilities offered by information technology to reduce these (p.37). It also speaks of constructing more 'bridges' between education, training and the labour market to allow for more complex and flexible trajectories than current parallel systems allow. This will clearly benefit all those women and men who do not follow the neat, ideal, male pattern of participation in education or training followed by work on a full-time basis until retirement. The conceptualisation of these 'pathways' is in terms of 'bringing marginalised groups *back* into the mainstream' (p.37) (my emphasis). This again indicates a conceptualisation of a hegemonic society from which these groups are excluded – creating more routes between education and training systems and the labour market is seen as the way to bringing them *back in*. As the model of exclusion propounded by Levitas suggests (1996), this reveals a dichotomised view of groups of insiders and outsiders and detracts attention from the inequalities between the educational, training and occupational lifechances of those already in employment: in particular it distracts attention from the needs of part-time and homeworkers, the vast majority of whom are women.

The idea of personal skill cards, which may have been influenced by the UK practice of accreditation of prior learning (APL), is about recognising and validating existing skills and offering potential employers a more up-to-date account of competences than certificates and diplomas which have been acquired some time ago, and which, given the short shelf-life of so many skills, may already be redundant. While there is no gendered discussion of personal skill cards, this policy, like APL, may well benefit women in particular, especially those returning to the labour market.

Hence, despite the lack of an explicit focus on women in the document beyond the exhortation to provide EO in a general sense, there are specific proposals which may be of particular benefit to women. Positive action, described in the document as positive discrimination (it is unclear which it is meant to be) is presented as an appropriate measure to combat social exclusion, in particular that of young urban youth. Women are not specifically identified as an 'excluded' group.

CONCLUSION

The spectre of street begging and young unemployed people becoming increasing disengaged from 'mainstream' society is clearly one that has influenced the drafting of the three EC White Papers which set the framework for the next decade on economic, social, education and training policy in the EU. Combating social exclusion is a leitmotiv which runs through all three. At the same time as seeking to generate a healthy, competitive, skill-based economy, there is a moral panic about social fragmentation. This is cast in terms of insiders and outsiders, a less cohesive and integrated society from which some souls have been excluded largely as a result of their lack of skills and therefore their inability to compete effectively for jobs.

The notion of equality expressed in the documents is couched in terms of equal treatment for men and women, and women as such are not defined as an excluded group. Nevertheless, gender is a significant discriminator of occupational lifechances. What the model of social exclusion obscures, as Levitas (1996) shows, is patent inequalities within the 'mainstream'. The impact of gender is downplayed, and inequality is couched in terms of lack of ability to compete effectively. However, a system based on competition will always have losers. The position of some of those losers is more obvious than that of others. The causes of variable rates of success in competition include systems and structures predicated on certain values and expectations of a dominant, culturally-determined gender contract.

The model of EO which underlines the policies is still based on treating individuals the same, irrespective of their gender, although positive action measures are clearly felt to be appropriate in certain circumstances. However, there is a failure to engage with the gendered nature of institutions and their structures and the impact of this on the distribution of opportunities. The emphasis is placed on helping those who perform less well within existing structures. This implies that existing structures are gender-neutral – which, of course, they are not. The current focus on social exclusion, then, while it may lead to policies and programmes which are of assistance to some, cannot but be limited in its achievements.

Positive action education and training projects, while welcome, only benefit a few and tend to be short-term. They do not affect the vast majority or challenge the practices of mainstream education and training provision. To make a significant difference, an EO approach has to recognise the androcentricity of existing provision and bring the equality agenda into mainstream provision. The White Papers do not address these issues, and therefore their success in achieving their aims will inevitably be highly limited. How could the equality agenda be 'mainstreamed'? This is the subject of the final chapter.

Chapter 10

Mainstreaming equality?

Men are the norm, women are 'other'.

(Simone de Beauvoir, 1949)

I dare say I am not the only person who experienced a frisson of voyeuristic delight on learning that Betty Boothroyd, our esteemed Speaker in the UK House of Commons, she who can control Government Ministers by raising one eyebrow, was in an earlier part of her life a Tiller Girl (Routledge 1996). The Tiller Girls, who graced our black-and-white television sets in the early 1960s, would perform high kicks while dancing in a line, arms linked behind their backs, wearing precarious and exotic headgear, and sporting the kind of genuine smiles which staff are now sent on customer service training courses to learn to emulate. What glamour! What precision! What synergy!

In a similar vein, I, too, can admit to engaging many years ago in an unlikely activity for an academic: as an undergraduate I was a drum majorette in the University Rag procession. Our 'squad' of twenty-one 19 to 20-year-old students was trained by a somewhat ill-matched pair of post-graduates: an army captain on secondment and a Californian ex-cheerleader. We learned to march in perfect time to the music and to twirl our batons while executing elaborate steps, some of which involved marching backwards no less. Indeed, our reputation spread and we were soon requested by other universities to lead their rag processions too. At one, we were awarded first prize in the competition for the best Rag 'float', despite a rather churlish challenge from a disgruntled rugby team as to our status as a 'float', given we were not performing on the back of a lorry. Nevertheless, this technical objection was overruled and we were duly presented with the first prize: eighty pints of free beer. As most of us only ventured as far as a Babycham at Christmas, this prize was of little interest, but we soon found our erstwhile challengers, having eventually gallantly admitted defeat, were all too keen to bury the hatchet and to befriend us for the evening.

I mention all this by way of evidence, of a kind, that women can synchronise with each other and, indeed, can march in routines far more complex than those usually demanded of a squaddie. This is significant when we consider that, of those would-be recruits to the armed services in the UK who undertake the initial six-week selection and training stage, women apparently outperform men in all the tests except one – marching.[1] They are much more likely to report problems with their pelvises incurred as a result of the daily rigours of marching. However (and this is the point of the story, for those who are getting concerned), this is because they are *marching to the male stride*. As men on the whole have longer legs than women, and as there are far more of them in the selection procedures for the armed services, it is the male stride which is adopted as the norm against which performance is measured. Women have difficulty in marching comfortably to the male stride. I see this as a metaphor for the first stage in the mainstreaming agenda: recognising that what is taken as the norm is not necessarily gender-neutral.

The essence of the mainstreaming approach is to seek to identify these hidden, unrecognised and unremarked ways in which systems and structures are biased in favour of men, and to redress the balance. It involves lateral thinking to see how apparently gender-neutral practices, which appear to offer equal access to all, in fact act as exclusionary mechanisms for women. And while the focus in this book has been on gender inequality, similar arguments and analyses could be presented for social construction of neutrality as norm on other equality dimensions, such as race and disability.

The book has been mostly concerned with training and with making the case for a mainstreaming approach towards EO within training policies and provision. However, training policies do not stand alone: they interact with policies and practices in education and the labour market. Their symbiotic relationship reinforces gendered trajectories whereby women and men are cemented into work places which are highly segregated horizontally, vertically, and by terms and conditions of employment. Gendered systems and structures characterise all three. Training could provide a challenge to these trends but is more likely to reinforce them. Equal treatment legislation has prompted some flexibility and positive action measures have provided women's spaces and the opportunity to develop good practice. However, for the most part, training systems, their mechanisms of funding, curricular (both formal and informal), pedagogy, models of the gendering of hierarchies, contact hours, ignoring of domestic commitments and so on, all serve to create opportunities structured by the differentials of the gender contract. What can mainstreaming offer here?

Mainstreaming has become a popularised slogan for a new approach to EO in the late 1990s. It is referred to as the main strategic approach for a range of national and international bodies. To recap, the European Commission's *Communication* to the Council of Ministers recommends incorporating EO into all Community actions, policies and programmes (CEC 1996). The United Nations Fourth World Conference on women in 1995 identified mainstreaming as one of its goals. In the UK, this resulted in mainstreaming being one of ten policy papers in the *National Agenda for Action* (Women's National Commission *et al.* 1996). The DfEE is piloting mainstreaming in all its internal and external activities (Birchard 1997) and other Government departments are showing an interest in following suit. The EOC has adopted mainstreaming as its main strategic approach to the development of EO in Britain (EOC 1996b).

Despite this high-level commitment, there are different accounts of what the concept means, and how it should be operationalised. The implication of mainstreaming for the future of positive action measures is contested. And its relationship with other human resource approaches, such as 'managing diversity', is far from clear. This chapter offers a view on some of these issues and seeks to provide clarification on areas of confusion. There is little doubt that, just like previous approaches to EO, such as those introduced in organisations studied by Cockburn (1991), there can be 'long and short' agendas simultaneously at play. The politics of EO are such that some hard-won ground can be undermined by recourse to the rhetoric of mainstreaming. In other words, organisations may believe, or wish it to be believed, that they are committed to EO, and introduce some measures to this end, but fall far short of the paradigm shift in thinking which would be required to make a more than superficial difference to the organisation's culture and praxis – and hence to women's education, training and occupational lifechances.

The emphasis in this account is on how mainstreaming could be conceptualised and what it might have to offer. The remarks are necessarily tentative. Despite the hyperbole and the rhetoric, the literature on mainstreaming is scant. And, notwithstanding the high profile support from influential national and international organisations for mainstreaming, there is as yet little empirical research. This is beginning to be addressed; there is, for example the EOC's transnational pilot project on mainstreaming in local government in four Member States, funded under the Fourth Medium Term Action Programme. However, it is as yet too early to assess what is being achieved in its name.

The chapter begins by addressing some of the conceptual ambiguities surrounding the concept of mainstreaming and, in particular, seeks to distance it from some of the tools that might be used in its implementation. In other words, it spells out what it is not, but what is sometimes passed off as mainstreaming. It goes on to examine the implications of gender contracts for how a mainstreaming approach might be delivered. It concludes with a prognostic account of how equal treatment, positive action and mainstreaming approaches (or, in my own formulation, tinkering, tailoring and transforming) might be brought together to create a paradigm shift in education, training and labour market policy.

WHAT IS MAINSTREAMING?

In conceptualising mainstreaming, I want to begin with what it is not. Gender impact studies, gender-proofing of documents, and gender monitoring, are all to my mind useful tools in a mainstreaming approach (although some reservations are expressed below about gender-proofing); but of themselves they will have little impact on policy development, implementation and outcome. Moreover, there is a danger that these tools may be seen as a substitute for the far more thoroughgoing and difficult approach which mainstreaming could and should be.

First of all, mainstreaming is not simply a 'gender impact' approach, where a policy is in essence 'vetted' for its likely impact on men and women. This approach, nevertheless, is a useful beginning and one which local authorities increasingly adopt in the process of reviewing policy developments, along with an environmental impact assessment. Indeed, gender impact studies are pressed for in the Platform for Action coming out of the UN Beijing Conference for the 'development, monitoring and

evaluation of all micro and macro economic and social policies'
(Section 167). Such an impact assessment might have led local
authorities to have anticipated that the fallout of compulsory
competitive tendering would be likely to lead to a systematic reduction in pay in female-dominated sectors, such as cleaning, already
characterised by low wages (Escott and Whitfield 1995). Hence,
although useful as a safety net in the absence of genuine mainstreaming, this approach is limited because it is *post hoc* and
reactive. Nevertheless, as a first step it can be effective as an awareness-raising exercise and sensitising device; it can train people to
think about policies in a different way, especially if it carries the
weight of law. In Sweden, for example, the Equality Affairs Division
of the Ministry of Health and Social Affairs has as one of its
responsibilities the duty 'to ensure that that the terms of reference
for government committees require them to analyse the gender
perspective in their work and the gender impact of any proposals
made' (EOC 1996b: 5). This review process is a necessary but not
sufficient part of mainstreaming, and there is a always a danger it
can become a 'tick and bash' procedure that does not command
serious attention if there are no sanctions to back it up or if the
Realpolitik means it can be safely ignored.

Gender-proofing of documents to check for sexist language and
sex-stereotyping in images is an indication of a concern that policy
may appear to be exclusive, but it may amount to no more than
window-dressing. Such an exercise does not necessarily address the
androcentric thinking behind such documents – indeed, it merely
obscures it. The criticism was made of the documentation relating
to the Action Programmes described in Chapter 7 that there was no
clear message on EO; indeed, the illustrations in FORCE material
reinforced gender stereotypes in relation to new technologies. The
absence of gender-proofing of policy documents, as in the White
Paper on Teaching and Learning discussed in Chapter 9 (EC
1996b), lays its androcentricity bare (although, in fairness, sexist
language not present in a document's original language is sometimes introduced in translation). While it is clearly important that
the discourse of policy documents is inclusive, and this is part of
the mainstreaming agenda, this should be the outcome of the
thinking behind it, rather than emerging as the result of a routine,
clerical checking procedure.

Gender-monitoring, where the gender composition of employees,
students, trainees, customers and so on can be compared with the

potential pool of recruits to gain insights into patterns of distortion, is essential in mainstreaming. However, once again, it is *post hoc*, and not all organisations which undertake gender-monitoring necessarily use the data in performance review and forward planning. The lack of gendered statistics which impeded the review of women in post-compulsory education and training in Wales was discussed in Chapter 5. More importantly, the lack of data showed that the TECs were ill-equipped to ensure that they were honouring their service-level agreements on EO for men and women, and, as we saw, this applied to their obligations on EO for ethnic minorities as well (Boddy 1995). The difficulties experienced by the EC in answering Madame Fontaine's question in the European Parliament about women's participation in the EC Action Programmes on education and training featured in Chapter 7, and in the following chapter, the problems associated with assessing the participation of women in ESF-funded activities were both due to the lack of statistical monitoring.

It is important to disaggregate statistics, not simply by gender, but by gender cross-tabulated with other variables to reveal the structural disadvantages experienced by smaller units of analysis, for example solo parents, members of specific ethnic minorities, or spatially specific areas undergoing industrial restructuring. The identification of appropriate units of analysis is key to the implementation of a mainstreaming agenda which is concerned about the inter-relationship among different equality dimensions. Many policies adopted in the name of gender equality, for example, have benefited well qualified, middle-class women with uninterrupted careers, but leave the vast majority of women untouched. This simply widens the pay gap between women, rather than closing the gap between women and men.

There is clearly much that could be done to improve our record-keeping, not simply at the organisational level but in terms of national and European-level statistics in this regard, if there were a political will to do so. For example, as long ago as 1983, *Statistics Sweden*, that country's national statistical service, began the task of ensuring that all statistics relating to individuals be collected and disaggregated by gender. Gender-disaggregated statistics can be an important tool in awareness-raising and provide a snapshot of the effect of policy on different groups. The UN Platform for Action makes the case for gender-disaggregated statistics for planning and evaluation (Section 209).

All these tools are valuable and serve a variety of purposes, from awareness-raising to policy review. However, they are all *post hoc*. Of themselves they have only indirect and circumscribed effects. The essence of mainstreaming is that EO thinking is integrated into the policy development process from the beginning. These tools are then valuable in supporting a mainstreaming approach, but of themselves they do not, to my mind, constitute mainstreaming. So, what do we mean by mainstreaming?

Mainstreaming entails a paradigm shift in thinking towards the development of policy and practice. It requires being able to see the ways in which current practice is gendered in its construction, despite appearing to be gender-neutral. This was exemplified in the example of marching to the male stride. Much of the taken-for-granted inequality needs to be questioned, such as the imbalance between the regularity with which resources are allocated to providing car parks for new factories but not workplace nurseries. Statistics can provide a starting point to understanding how disadvantage is structured. The analysis of discourse, as we saw in Chapter 5, can also reveal androcentric biases in the social construction of concepts such as skill. Positive action projects, such as those described at various junctures in this book, have made a considerable contribution in developing good practice which is woman-centred in its curricula, pedagogy, organisational management and so on. As Lefebvre (1993) notes, what are seen as 'accompanying measures' in positive action for women, both 'upstream' (EO training awareness for employers) and 'downstream' (guidance, access, childcare support), need to be integrated into standard provision because they are so vital to a substantial proportion of consumers of training. Moreover, as various studies have shown, there is a growing view that practice which accommodates difference can make good business sense (Rubery and Humphries 1995).

GENDER CONTRACTS

The limitations of EO policies in bringing about significant change in patterns of gender segregation have been well documented (Cockburn 1991, Coyle 1995). Jewson *et al.* (1995), on the basis of their research, outline five models of the articulation of EO with employment policy and practice: serendipity (an *ad hoc* approach); dissociation (formal policies but without systematic implementation); accommodation (EO practice consolidated around a formal policy but lacking strategic thinking and systematic followthrough); integration (comprehensive pro-active EO practices focused on a detailed and ongoing formal policy); and assimilation (absorption of EO policy and implementation into business strategies and routines).

It is the last of these which comes closest to mainstreaming, and in this formulation has many resonances of 'managing diversity', another ill-defined and much over-used concept. Conceptual work by Liff (1996) illustrates the tensions between conventional approaches to EO and managing diversity. She argues that it is important to differentiate between level of commitment to equality and perceived relevance of gender differentiation to the organisation. Within this framework, models of EO and managing diversity can share similarities as well as exhibit differences. Empirical work by Kandola and Fullerton (1994) present other models of managing diversity which move beyond gender to accommodate other differences. The difficulty which emerges in both is the issue of valuing difference.

Jewson et al.'s (1995) assimilation model, and managing diversity and mainstreaming approaches, carry the inherent danger that by becoming everything they become nothing. Meanwhile the 'special' safeguards of EO, such as equality officers, units and so on, may be dismantled in the name of mainstreaming. The model's authors point out how in this model, the emphasis shifts from groups and distributive justice to individuals and their self-realisation. And yet, even if issues of structural and cultural disadvantage were to be tackled successfully at the plant or organisational level, this begs the question of the wider culture within which the organisation and its employees (or students, or trainees) operate. This brings us back to the subject of gender contracts.

One of the major reason for the limitations of EO policies has been the wider culture within which the organisation is situated, and the inter-relationship between education, training and employment referred to above. All three are undergoing change, some at a faster rate than others. For example, the education system of Spain has had a major overhaul, Finland is experiencing new, high levels of unemployment, and the economies of Eastern European countries, many of which may well soon become members of the EU, are undergoing dramatic restructuring. These shifts impact upon the nature of the gender contract. So we see that one of the impacts of unemployment on the new Länder of Germany is to challenge women's status as legitimate members of the workforce, especially when unemployed. The gender contract of the old Länder is being imposed on the new.

There are continuities, too, however. Some case studies of organisational culture have managed to capture the impact, or rather lack of impact, of some of the changes in work practices on women. Coyle (1995), for example, examined five contrasted case studies of UK employers with a view to assessing the impact of organisational change on women's employment opportunities. She reviewed whether the EO policies in operation at the companies concerned were appropriate to the new conditions and whether they were integral to the management of change. She concluded (1995: ix):

> Equal opportunity employment policies have not been without impact. They have undoubtedly helped the progression of individual women and they have helped place a whole range of new issues onto the workplace agenda. It is important that employers are urged to continue with such policies. However, equal opportunity policies have not achieved any significant change in patterns of gendered occupational segregation and pay differentials. The new labour market conditions of the late 1990s indicate the need for new actions and new actors in the equality project. The feminisation of work and explosive growth of temporary, part-time and low paid work has implications for men as well as women. It has implications for family income, job insecurity and even the housing market, pension and social policy. Broad based issues such as equal pay for work of equal value, rights for part-time and temporary workers, working hours and the care of children and the elderly are scarcely new. These are concerns that women have long highlighted. What is new is that these issues are increasingly of relevance to men. The scope for common cause on the basis of a more transformative equal opportunities agenda should perhaps now be examined.

It is here we see the link being made between internal (organisation-specific) EO policies and the reality of external gender relations. It is only if all policies, housing, welfare, tax, pensions and so on, take on board the need to treat individuals as individuals rather than as gendered members of nuclear families that mainstreaming policies in education, training and the labour market can begin to have some purchase. This is why the EC's Communication to the Council of Ministers recommending the incorporation of EO into all Community action policies and programmes is, potentially at least (there is no guarantee whatsoever that it will be heeded), a very powerful document.

However, it is also dangerous, in the same way that Jewson *et al.* (1995) describe assimilation as 'potentially Janus-faced'. For, while patriarchal relations continue to govern educational, training and occupational lifechances, dismantling EO safeguards, despite their limited effectiveness, would be highly risky and retrogressive. Moreover, the eradication of patriarchal relations, inequalities as a result of ethnic origin and so on, is an extremely long-term agenda. Mainstreaming policies, unless accompanied by more traditional EO polices based on a recognition of difference, may well be counter-productive.

In sum, equal treatment legislation needs to continue alongside further development of positive action measures while the mainstreaming approach is developed. Far more strategic approaches need to be developed to graft onto the good practices learned from positive action into mainstream provision. Meanwhile, developing awareness through gender-disaggregated statistics, routine gender-monitoring, and gender impact assessments of new policies across the board, will start to address the gender contract agenda. The male breadwinner/female homemaker model needs to be replaced with a new gender contract that allows for greater equality between men and women. This means nothing less than a complete rethink of how the gender contract is underpinned in systems and structures, and an overhaul of all legislation.

An approach along these lines has been attempted in Sweden. State policy between 1960 and 1975 sought to replace the breadwinner/homemaker gender contract with what Hirdmann (1990) describes as a double income 'equality' gender contract. Higher female economic activity rates followed; however, new patterns of gender segregation emerged within the workplace. Indeed, women are largely found in the service sector which is now severely threatened by public expenditure cuts. Since the late 1970s, however, a new gender contract era emerged, described by Hirdmann as the 'equal status contract', in which women and men should share not simply employment opportunities but also domestic responsibilities and family care. This allows much more freedom of choice for men as well as women to identify personal strategies to balance home and work.

There is a variety of contractual arrangements which allow this balance to be achieved. This is brought out in Hobson's (1997) work on solo mothers in five Member States. She identifies two ideal models of state-supported gender contract arrangements for care services. The 'Parent Worker' model, which approximates most closely to that adopted in Sweden, entitles the caretaking parent(s) to care services for dependants so that they can engage in the labour market full-time. By contrast, the 'Caregiving Social Wage Model', which comes close to the system in the Netherlands, assumes all mothers will be carers and, therefore, in the absence of a bread-winner, provides solo mothers with a social wage for their caring services. Both recognise the importance of care work, and both help to avoid the poverty experienced by solo mothers in other Member States such as the USA, Germany (before reunification) and the UK. By helping solo mothers to avoid poverty, these models facilitate women wanting to invest in their own human capital. This is in contrast to the UK where many solo mothers, with inadequate access to childcare and living at subsistence level for a prolonged period, have very little opportunity to take up their opportunities for 'equal access' to training.

The Swedish experience does not mean a new reality overnight, and the gains are precarious. Nevertheless, this approach includes the systematic scrutiny, from an EO perspective, of all proposals for government legislation before discussion in cabinet (EOC 1996b). This comes very close to mainstreaming equality, as it tackles the issue of gender contracts across the board and at an early stage in the planning process. It is more far-reaching than EO measures categorised earlier as tinkering or tailoring – or indeed those activities (such as gender monitoring) which are a necessary but not sufficient component of mainstreaming. Within a context of universal scrutiny from a gendered perspective, there is the potential for mainstreaming equality within education, training and the labour market to have more impact.

This brings me back to the three White Papers discussed in Chapter 9 on economic, social and teaching/learning policy in the EU, and to what I see as the fundamental contradiction that underlies them. The intention to offer equal treatment to men and women (as enshrined in the Treaty of Rome) is juxtaposed with that of creating opportunities for competition between individuals within a system based upon gendered constructions of 'merit'. This is a confusion of acknowledged group-based disadvantage and championing of individual competition within rules that clearly favour specific groups (hence the acknowledgement of, and intention to address, the problem of 'socially excluded groups'). The failure to recognise the significance of gender in the analysis of the challenges to be faced in the economic White Paper (1994a), so roundly criticised by the 'seven wise women' (EC 1995d), indicates a 'gender-neutral' interpretation of a highly gendered labour market, while accepting a particular form of gender contract (breadwinner/homemaker) as a given rather than an ideological social construction underpinned by both national and European systems. This contradiction is repeated in the Teaching and Learning White Paper (EC 1996b), while the Social Policy White Paper (EC 1994b) openly acknowledges that women (and their children) are especially likely to be among the socially excluded. No connection is made between these positions, and yet it is clear that, if women are in an equal position 'to compete', they would not need to be on the receiving end of special treatment for the disadvantaged. The rules of competition are drawn up to favour men. Women who are unable to march to the male stride are anticipated as casualties of social exclusion, but without the acknowledgement that it is the stride, rather than their marching, which is the cause.

CONCLUSION

This book set out to make a contribution to the enduring debate about the mechanisms which perpetuate patterns of gender segregation in the labour market, despite changes in social climate, legislation, new technologies, skill shortages and the restructuring of the labour market. The emphasis has been on the part training systems and structures play in the reproduction of gender segregation.

At the same time, the book gives an account of the EC's approaches to EO, tracing a shift from equal treatment to positive action, and the current policy of mainstreaming (tinkering, tailoring and transforming). It is argued that mainstreaming, while gaining an ascendancy in many national and international policy arenas, is poorly conceptualised and inadequately understood. Competing definitions co-exist. Moreover, there is a danger that many of the hard-won mechanisms which are designed to shore up EO may be dismantled in the name of mainstreaming. Nevertheless, while mindful of these dangers, and of the fact that mainstreaming is a very long-term agenda, it has the potential to deliver more than previous models of EO described and critiqued here. It needs to address the fundamental issue of gender contracts in order to make a significant difference to women's education, training and occupational opportunities.

In essence, the mainstreaming agenda has to tackle head-on the complexities of the relationship between capital and patriarchy, and how these are manifested in gender contracts. The OECD (1994) has taken a lead in arguing that education, training and labour market policies need to be harmonised with caring, taxation and welfare systems to enable individuals to operate as individuals as well as family members. The ideology of the white nuclear family underpins so many of our social institutions, despite the fact that this leads to systematic disadvantage for women, resulting in their being undervalued and experiencing destitution in old age because of a labour market geared to men. The White Papers begin to address some of the rigidities in VET systems in the context of an ageing workforce, growing unemployment and the exigencies of the information society.

The concern about women, as Europe's poor and as the unskilled section of a workforce that needs to be flexible and skilled, creates a climate whereby these issues might be tackled. There is also a widespread concern about skill shortages, economic competitiveness and unemployment. In each of these areas, women's training needs are also those of the EU. Politically, the Commissioners currently responsible for the EO brief include some whose sophistication in understanding these issues and commitment to EO is far more developed than that of any predecessor. The impact of Dr Monika Wulf-Matheis (European Commissioner responsible for Regional Affairs) on the EFDF is already being felt; Commissioner Anita Gradin comes with a wealth of experience of mainstreaming from Sweden. However, other forces are also coming into play, and there are losses as well as gains, as the women of the former German Democratic Republic are experiencing as their own gender contract is replaced by that of the former Federal Republic of Germany. And while there may be a political will to move some way towards mainstreaming in terms of gender equality, however defined, there are, as yet, few signs of moving beyond it to embrace other forms of inequality.

Directorates-General of the European Commission

I	External Economic Relations
IA	External Political Relations
II	Economic and Financial Affairs
III	Industrial Affairs
IV	Competition
V	Employment, Industrial Relations and Social Affairs
VI	Agriculture
VII	Transport
VIII	Development
IX	Personnel and Administration
X	Information, Communication, Culture and Audio-visual Media
XI	Environment, Nuclear Safety and Civil Protection
XII	Science, Research and Development
XIII	Telecommunications, Information Market and Exploitation of Research
XIV	Fisheries
XV	Internal Market and Financial Services
XVI	Regional Policy and Cohesion
XVII	Energy
XVIII	Credit and Investments
XIX	Budgets
XX	Financial Control
XXI	Customs and Indirect Taxation
XXII	Education, Training and Youth
XXIII	Enterprise Policy, Distributive Trades, Tourism and Cooperatives
XXIV	Consumer Policy

National Vocational Qualifications

Level 1 Competence which involves the application of knowledge in the performance of a range of varied work activities, most of which may be routine or predictable.

Level 2 Competence which involves the application of knowledge in a significant range of varied work activities, performed in a variety of contexts. Some of the activities are complex or non-routine and there is some individual responsibility and autonomy. Collaboration with others, perhaps through membership of a work group or team, may often be a requirement.

Level 3 Competence which involves the application of knowledge in a broad range of varied work activities performed in a wide variety of contexts, most of which are complex and non-routine. There is considerable responsibility and autonomy, and control or guidance of others is often required.

Level 4 Competence which involves the application of knowledge in a broad range of complex technical or professional work activities performed in a wide variety of contexts and with a substantial degree of personal responsibility and autonomy. Responsibility for the work of others and the allocation of resources is often present.

Level 5 Competence which involves the application of a significant range of fundamental principles across a wide and often unpredictable variety of contexts. Very substantial personal autonomy and often significant responsibility for the work of others and for the allocation of substantial resources feature strongly, as do personal accountabilities for analysis and diagnosis, design, planning execution and evaluation.

Commission of the European Communities

SEC(93) 1977; Brussels, 3 December 1993

Social Dialogue Joint Opinion on Women and Training

INTRODUCTION

Vocational education and training is recognised by the Social Partners as one of the key elements to the success of the Single Market. In an increasingly competitive market, it is vital to have a highly skilled workforce in order to avoid skill gaps and to counteract potential labour shortages.[1] As the Social Partners already stated in a previous Joint Opinion,[2] 'completion of the internal market strengthens the case for increasing investment in and access to training and improving the quality and quantity of training measures'. Given that women are playing an ever-increasing role in the economic and social development of the European Community, it is important to improve and develop where necessary their vocational education and training on an equal footing with men so that they can contribute fully to the success of the Single Market.

In the Joint Opinion on Education and Training (19 June 1990), the Social Partners have already proposed that 'policies promoting equal opportunities for men and women and, in particular, the participation of women in all training schemes, especially those linked to the occupations of the future, should be developed and specific measures should be devised as regards training for occupations in which women are under-represented'. In this Joint Opinion, the Social Partners wish to further advance proposals to improve the vocational skills of women through education and training.

Considerable improvements have been made to legislative provision concerning equal treatment for women in vocational training and employment opportunities in the European Community in recent years. Legal rights and protection for women have been extended. Furthermore, there is ample empirical evidence that women's participation in the labour market has increased and that their career opportunities have improved in the EC over the last decades. There is also a trend towards diversification of girls' vocational choices which improves their prospect on the labour market.

These positive developments and trends need to be accelerated and reinforced by complementary action focused on specific target groups who need special support. Public authorities, including educational institutions and training organisations at all levels, as well as employers and trade unions, have an important role to play in this respect. The media has also a significant contribution to make in this respect.

It is important to recognise that the position of women in the labour market is strongly influenced by cultural attitudes which prevail in society in general but in particular in families, education, enterprises and trade unions. These cultural attitudes still result in both structural and attitudinal barriers to women's integration in the labour market. On the one hand, outdated assumptions by parents, teachers, employers and trade unions about the role of women in society can limit women's expectations of their potential career opportunities. On the other hand, both the care of children and adult dependants, as long as they remain essentially the responsibility of women, put structural constraints on women's labour market participation and career progression. Furthermore, while there is no legal discrimination in access to training for women, the Social Partners acknowledge that in practice women do not participate equally with men in vocational training and believe that they can play an important role in promoting open-minded and positive attitudes and behaviour towards women on the labour market and in society.

While recognising the scope and complexity of the issues involved, the Social Partners acknowledge their responsibility in supporting employment and training policies, both in the workplace and outside, that will secure gains for women by opening up wider training and career development opportunities.

There is a series of pressing arguments for a focus on women and training in the decade to come.

Demographic changes imply that, in the long run, there will be insufficient young people entering the labour market to meet demand. It is also the case that, numerically, women will be a highly significant group in the labour force of the 1990s. They already constitute the majority of the new job holders and new labour market entrants in the Community.[3] They also comprise the majority of the unemployed, and the principal source of untapped available labour supply in the future. Providing opportunities for women and encouraging them to improve and diversify their professional qualifications will contribute to ensure the necessary equilibrium between supply and demand in the labour market. Women's participation at all levels and in all sectors of the economy will also contribute to greater balance in every aspect of life.

As a consequence, it is vital that public authorities, the Social Partners and other actors, each according to their own responsibilities, enable and encourage all such categories of women to participate in relevant initial and continuing vocational training, e.g.:

• those entering the labour market for the first time,
• those in employment at all levels, regardless of legal status, including temporary, part-time and fixed-term contract workers,
• unemployed women,
• women returners,
• women in rural areas.

Nowadays, in most European countries, women generally obtain a high level of educational achievement although in a more limited range of subjects than men. In spite of efforts having been made to diversify women's vocational choices and thereby improve their integration into the labour market, women are still mainly trained and employed in either low-skilled occupations or in areas of skilled employment predominated by women. Resulting from this, their opportunities are often limited to female dominated sectors.[4] Women's professional choices are limited by this clustering in female dominated sectors. Greater progress needs to be made by schools, public authorities, enterprises and trade unions, each according to their own responsibility, in providing opportunities and in encouraging girls and women so that they participate in education and training for occupations which give them access to a wider range of future oriented, high-skilled employment.

The need for the EC's economies to undergo industrial restructuring in order to gain in competitiveness means that there will need to be a smooth reallocation of workers from surplus to deficit sectors: this will be essential for a successful economy. Gender segregation based on vocational orientation contributes to a major labour market rigidity. It impedes the smooth reallocation of workers and contributes to unnecessary unemployment, short-term skills mismatches and longer-term skills gaps. Special training support is necessary to overcome this segregation.[5]

In this context, it is necessary to adopt an innovative approach to the participation of women in general education and vocational training activities, including in enterprise-based training programmes. This approach must respond to the varying attitudes, abilities, motivations, expectations and cultural experiences on the part of women themselves and provide training appropriate to their respective needs and to the needs of the market. Improving the skills of women in the labour market, through vocational training, will contribute to the promotion of equality of opportunity in the workplace, as well as to the better use of human resources.

Finally, the Social Partners would like to call on all actors, including women themselves, to assume their own responsibility with regard to existing initial and continuing training opportunities.

LINES OF APPROACH

1 The Social Partners believe that the skills potential of women should be maximised as a labour market resource.
2 Women's participation and position in the labour market are not determined solely by economic factors but are also influenced by cultural attitudes. Therefore, the Social Partners consider that there is a need to promote cultural and social change to ensure a positive and progressive environment.
3 The Social Partners support measures, at all appropriate levels, which would allow women to participate under the same conditions as men in vocational education and training investment aimed at upskilling the labour force.
4 The Social Partners agree to work towards encouraging full participation and integration of women into all occupational areas and levels. This will facilitate a more beneficial use of human resources. Training as a means of improving access opportunities for women to employment and promotion opportunities for women is not only compatible with but essential for the economic advance of the European Community.
5 The Social Partners believe that innovative measures should be taken, both inside and outside the workplace, particularly in schools, to diversify vocational choice among girls and women by means of guidance measures directed towards a wider range of future-oriented careers. Measures should be taken to encourage

participation on an equal footing of women and men in education and training programmes, thereby improving their opportunities for greater participation at all levels of the enterprise.

6 The Social Partners consider that this overall approach needs to be underpinned by a wide range of positive support initiatives to include care of dependants and where necessary further publicity campaigns to increase general awareness.

7 In order to achieve lasting success in women's vocational diversification, all those concerned, including employers and workers and their representatives, should take the necessary steps to facilitate the integration of women in enterprises which still have a predominantly male workforce today.

RECOMMENDATIONS

1 Member States and the Community should continue and develop positive strategies to promote women's training, leading to a wider range of employment opportunities and career progression.

2 In order to ensure greater transparency and matching of women's skills with labour market demand, the Social Partners recommend to the Community and public authorities that steps should be taken to compile existing relevant information and, where necessary, to provide further information about labour market prospects and training possibilities for women. Such information should cover both the different levels in the Member States and the Community programmes. Attention should be paid to special target groups, e.g. women returners to the labour market, and unemployed women who need to change their vocational orientation.

3 Measures should be taken to promote access on an equal footing for women and men to vocational training. It has been observed in many cases that the appropriate choice of the selection criteria applied and the resources made available for training programmes have increased access of women to vocational training. The Social Partners recommend that such practices be encouraged and developed at all levels, within private and public enterprises, at local, regional, national and Community levels.

4 The Social Partners recommend that, in the design of training programmes, due consideration should be given to the need for

women and men to combine work and family responsibilities. In this context, the appropriate use of open and distance learning programmes combined with support at local level should be examined.

5 The Social Partners wish to explore ways in which the role of SMEs in vocational education and training can be enhanced, e.g. through the use of incentives.

6 A compendium of examples of good practice should be compiled at Community level based on an analysis of valuable experience gained across the Community. This compendium should be developed within the framework of an *ad hoc* group under the supervision of the Social Dialogue and be directed at providers of education and training and policymakers at all levels.

7 At Community level, urgent steps should be taken to ensure greater coherence, transparency and better coordination between Community funded programmes contributing to the training of women, both in the TFRH and in the Social Fund, including effective monitoring and evaluation procedures.

There should be a periodic publication of a simple guide to all the potential Community sources for funding of women's training. Information should be provided on access to such programmes. Particular efforts should be made to ensure that the projects funded comply with established non-discriminatory selection criteria which effectively lead to an improvement in the occupational position of women.

8 As part of the process of cultural change affecting both men and women, the Social Partners recommend that:

- gender prejudice be eliminated from subject choice and teaching methods (e.g. school textbooks) in educational establishments;
- trainers and managers be made aware of potential barriers to the integration of girls and women into a wider range of technical and future orientated occupations, where necessary through the introduction of specific modules concerning relevant legislation;
- the media should also contribute to this cultural change.

9 In addition to the recommendations already set out in Joint Opinions,[6] the Social Partners wish to draw attention to certain issues of particular importance for the training of women.

School curricula should provide a broad basic education which enables girls and boys to make career choices based on the full range of employment opportunities. An effective and well-resourced vocational guidance service including a European dimension should be available to all pupils.

10 Effective counselling and guidance facilities need to be provided in order that women, as well as men, at all stages of their education and working lives should have complete and up-to-date information about training and employment prospects. This should be undertaken through further cooperation between the Social Partners and all the relevant institutions and should also involve the European Commission.

11 Measures and initiatives to advance training and employment opportunities for women so that they are on equal footing with men need to continue at all levels. Further progress needs to be made in advancing mainstream training opportunities for women workers.

In the context of the European Social Fund, the Social Partners strongly recommend the continuation of specific measures targeted at women with special needs (e.g. women returners, unemployed women undergoing retraining). The Social Partners also recommend measures that guarantee much greater participation by women in co-financed ESF mainstream programmes. The same consideration and recommendations apply to other EC education and training programmes, including qualifications initiatives.

12 The Social Partners note that many initiatives, including agreements in some Member States, have been developed concerning vocational training opportunities for women. They welcome these initiatives and recommend that this approach be extended further where appropriate. Existing evaluation studies of these initiatives should be compiled and analysed at European level in order to provide a basis for discussions about good practice and for further initiatives to be developed throughout the European Community.

13 The Social Partners agree to follow progress on issues concerning women's vocational education and training resulting from this Joint Opinion.

Equal treatment and positive action in LEONARDO DA VINCI
Guidelines for project promoters

1 EQUAL ACCESS PROJECTS

All projects open to both men and women should specify what measures they will adopt to ensure equal access as part of their EO objectives, particularly those in areas where one or other sex is under-represented. While it is recognised that seeking to ensure that men and women are offered equal access cannot guarantee that equal numbers of men and women will participate, imaginative pro-active methods of encouraging equal access can contribute towards breaking down stereotyping. Moreover, projects can include much broader EO objectives, such as seeking to ensure that the curriculum, pedagogy and materials are appropriate for both men and women, promoting training to encourage men and women in areas more traditionally associated with the opposite sex or offering gender-specific role models and mentors.

Promoters should also consider the EO dimensions of their internal organisation and hierarchy and state whether they have an EO policy.

Projects should seek to integrate where appropriate what have been called 'supplementary measures' to address women's training needs, such as counselling, confidence-building and de-stereotyping. Similarly, attention should be given in the design of proposals to the Commission's concern for the balance of home and working life, by addressing issues of childcare and family responsibilities of participants and providers.

The specific implications for promoters of equal access projects of the policy on mainstreaming EO is as follows:

- take steps to encourage participation by both sexes, if necessary by using innovative means;

- monitor participation by gender, both of consumers (e.g. trainees) and providers (e.g. project staff);
- ensure project materials are appropriate for both sexes;
- ensure curriculum and pedagogy are appropriate for both sexes.

2 POSITIVE ACTION PROJECTS

There is provision in LEONARDO DA VINCI for specific positive action projects for women and men to combat existing inequalities (measures I.1.d and II.1.d). Promoters with a positive action project in mind should pay attention to the following elements:

- the need to define the target group in detail (e.g. 'women' is too broad a group);
- the need to define in detail the development of new methodologies/pedagogics/materials, where appropriate;
- the importance of considering how the results and lessons of the project could be fed back into mainstream provision through the design of a dissemination programme. This might include production and dissemination of materials, monitoring and evaluation reports, linked research projects and presentation at seminars and conferences and so on. Any specific plans to work with target audiences are important here.
- the need to identify the likely value-added of the project for mainstreaming EO in the longer term.

Examples of equal treatment, positive action and mainstreaming in LEONARDO DA VINCI projects

The following examples of model projects have been designed to illustrate the differences between equal treatment, positive action and mainstreaming approaches to equal opportunities. They are arranged under the priority themes for 1996.

1 ACQUISITION OF NEW SKILLS

Strand I example: Training for people wanting to become self-employed or set up their own businesses

Equal treatment

A transnational project which offers training in setting up business to men and women, targeting the unemployed.

Positive action

A project which recognises that many women returning to work after a period of childcare who want to become self-employed or set up their own businesses may lack confidence, need childcare facilities, only be available at certain times of the day, not have previous business experience and be mystified by business jargon. They may also have poor access to start-up funds and only be interested in working on a part-time basis. Transnational projects can show up similarities and differences in approach, providing learning opportunities.

A positive action project would start from these concerns. It would seek to demystify the jargon by relating 'cash-flow', for example, to household budgeting skills. The training would be available at suitable hours and venues for women. Role models and mentors could be used.

Mainstreaming

A mainstreaming approach would seek to embed good practice in business support training for women into mainstream provision. The target group in this approach is more likely to be business agency support staff. Transnational working could assist the development of materials featuring a variety of potential entrepreneurs rather than stereotypes. The issues of particular concern to women, such as confidence-building, mentoring, childcare and not being taken seriously, need to be addressed as routine practice. Follow-on work, using structural funds, could involve development work with finance houses to encourage them to recognise women as good risks, and with ethical funding agencies wanting to invest in businesses in particular localities, regions or sectors.

2 LINKS BETWEEN VOCATIONAL AND EDUCATIONAL INSTITUTIONS AND ENTERPRISES

Strand II example: Transnational work placements for engineering students

Equal treatment

Short placements for final-year degree course engineering students in companies in three Member States to gain European level experience. Open to both male and female students.

Positive action

Placement for female students in companies which are 'women-friendly', that is, they already employ some women engineers and operate 'family-friendly' policies.

Mainstreaming

The research evidence suggests that many qualified women drop out of engineering not because of the work but because of what they experience as an oppressive, male-dominated work culture. A mainstreaming project which sought to tackle this issue would bring together Social Partners, equality agencies and researchers at the transnational level to develop ideas on how the male culture and work environment of engineering plants could be made more 'woman-friendly', and how employment practices could become more 'family-friendly'.

3 COMBATING SOCIAL EXCLUSION

Strand I example: outreach work with disaffected youth

Equal treatment

A project aimed at networking outreach initiatives which seek to encourage school truants and unemployed school-leavers with no qualifications to invest in their skill development. The aim of the project is to learn from and disseminate good practice and to offer such young people the opportunity for exchanges. Open to young men and women.

Positive action

A similar project but one that targets young women.

Mainstreaming

A project which seeks to discover and disseminate best practice at the transnational level in accommodating the specific training needs of young women, including teenage mothers, within outreach projects for disaffected youth.

4 PROMOTING INVESTMENT IN HUMAN RESOURCES

Strand III example: development of multimedia tools in sector-specific human resource management

Equal treatment

A project which brings together human resource experts from large companies and personnel organisations in Member States to develop multimedia tools on good human resource management in specific sectors, which includes an equal opportunities section.

Positive action

A similar project, but one which focuses in particular on developing expertise in equal opportunities.

Mainstreaming

A project which integrates equal opportunities into all the sections on human resource management good practice.

5 THE INFORMATION SOCIETY AND LIFELONG LEARNING

Strand III example: development of packages for training in computing skills for pre-release prisoners

Equal treatment

The project is designed to develop multimedia, self-directed learning computer packages for pre-release prisoners to develop computing skills, to ease their transition to working life on release. The package will be developed for and made available to both men and women prisoners.

Positive action

Given that women tend to have particular fears about new technologies, especially those of mature age who have not learned about them in school, the packages will be designed especially for women, and feature women as examples in the materials. They will seek to reinforce and build confidence and use problem-solving approaches which research suggests are more effective for women's learning styles.

Mainstreaming

A mainstreaming approach would integrate knowledge about gender-specific learning styles into the design of the packages, offering choices in ways to learn. Attention would be paid to 'gender-proofing' the materials throughout.

Notes

1 INTRODUCTION

1 The European Economic Community (EEC) was preceded by the European Coal and Steel Community which was set up in 1952. The Treaty of Rome then established the EEC in 1957. After the Maastricht Treaty in 1994, the EEC became the European Union (EU). Throughout the book I have referred to the EEC as covering the period 1957–1994 and the EU to refer to the post-1994 period.

    The European Commission (EC) is the civil service of the EU and is more pro-active in proposing policy than that of the UK. It will be noted in the references that pre-Maastricht Treaty Commission documents are described as coming from the Commission of the European Communities (CEC), while most (but not all) of those published after 1992 are referenced as European Commission (EC). I have followed the wording on the documents concerned in all cases.

2 The issue of how gender segregation should be measured over time and transnationally is a strongly contested one. Janet Siltanen refers to it as the 'housework' of gender segregation research. She and her colleagues have criticised two of the most commonly used indices, the Index of Dissimilarity and the Organisation for Economic Cooperation and Development's WE Index, and have developed their own, more sophisticated model (Blackburn *et al.* 1993). This model itself, however, has also been the subject of criticism (Lampard 1994; Watts 1994) which has been roundly rebutted (Blackburn *et al.* 1994a, 1994b).

3 See Appendix 1 for a full list of the Directorate-Generals of the European Commission

2 THE CONTEXT

1 In the UK, there are unique restrictions regarding eligibility for Job Seekers' Allowance for certain categories of married women and for those seeking part-time employment.

2 The emphasis on the low labour costs of Pacific rim countries in the White Paper is rather paradoxical in the light of the decision of LG

(Lucky Goldstar), the Korean company, to develop the largest inward investment project ever known in Europe in Newport, Wales, promising the creation of 6,000 jobs, on the grounds (*inter alia*) that wage rates were lower in Wales than in Korea. The size of grants provided by the Welsh Office, which was undoubtedly a key factor, is not being revealed to the public. It is also clear that a base within the Single Market is attractive to Pacific rim countries for trading purposes.

3 The text of the Social Partners' *Joint Opinion on Women and Training* (CEC/Social Dialogue 1993) is reproduced in Appendix III.

3 CONCEPTUALISING EQUAL OPPORTUNITIES

1 These linguistic and cultural variations in terms and their meanings are not, of course, confined to EO issues but characterise other transnational debates, such as training. 'Alternance' has become a universal 'European' word to describe a mixture of on- and off-the-job training in the absence of a convenient alternative in many languages. When I attended the meetings of the Social Partners preparing their *Joint Opinion on Women and Training* in 1992/3 (see Appendix III), some of the differences in understanding of EO and other terms emerged in debate: where terms did not exist in all the (then) Community languages, reference to them was avoided in the text. This raises for English speakers, of course, the intriguing question of what terms and concepts are available in other languages but not necessarily in English. In the absence of a term for key concepts in some languages, translators and interpreters may reach for the nearest logical equivalent, which may be wide of the mark. In my own rather unfortunate experience of German simultaneous interpretation in a presentation in Berlin, my use of the term 'manpower' (as in 'Manpower Services Commission') was rendered 'male virility'.

2 The EOC covers England, Scotland and Wales. There is also an EOC Northern Ireland which was set up under separate legislation.

3 It should be remembered that boys in some parts of the country, such as Manchester, benefited from a quota system designed to ensure that equal numbers of boys and girls had a grammar school education to counterbalance the fact that more girls than boys scored highly in the eleven-plus examination. This seems to have been forgotten in the current furore about 'under-achieving' boys.

4 In the UK, there are restrictions on married women gaining access to certain training provision for the unemployed (see EOC 1993).

5 Tinkering, tailoring and transforming appear to defy translation: they tend to be rendered as '*le tinkering, le tailoring, et le transforming*' in EC publications that have been translated.

6 The extent to which gender monitoring is used by Training and Enterprise Councils and training providers in England and Wales is discussed in Chapter 5.

4 THE EUROPEAN UNION AND EQUAL OPPORTUNITIES

1 Commissioner Flynn was a minister in the Irish Government when the decision was made not to allow a 13-year-old rape victim the opportunity to have an abortion.

2 Gender segregation is, of course, a feature of the European Commission itself. A recent publication shows how women represent 45 per cent of the staff of the Commission, but, among top officials (categories A1 and A2), there only five women compared with over two hundred men. There is a trend towards a better balance of women in top grades but from a very low base line. The EC has set up an Equal Opportunities Committee (COPEC) and two positive action programmes for female staff (1988–90 and 1992–96) (EC 1994c).

3 Article 189 of the Treaty of Rome provides that:

> In order to carry out their task the Council and Commission shall, in accordance with the provisions of the Treaty, make regulations, issue directives, take decisions, make recommendations or deliver opinions.

> A *Directive* is binding upon the Member States to which it is addressed, but leaves it to the national authorities to choose the form and methods of implementation. A *Regulation* is binding in its entirety and directly applicable to Member States. A *Decision* is binding in its entirety upon those to whom it is addressed. *Commission Recommendations* and *Council Opinions* have no binding force, but indicate policy directions.

4 For a detailed accounts of the ECJ and its impact on EO, see Nielson and Szyszczak (1991) and Meehan (1993). The work of the Network of Experts on the Implementation of the Equality Directives is described in a series of reports published by DGV – see, for example, Prechal and Senden (1994).

5 KEY ISSUES IN WOMEN'S EDUCATION AND TRAINING IN THE UK

1 A recent review of those employers taking positive action measures under the Act showed that they tended to employ a thousand employees or more, and that their main reason for introducing positive action for ethnic minorities was to demonstrate a commitment to social justice and make better use of human resources (Welsh *et al.* 1994). The Commission for Racial Equality has addressed the issue of Training and Enterprise Councils and racial equality through some of its publications (Commission for Racial Equality 1991, 1992).

2 The 'Ruskin debate' was so called in reference to a speech by then Prime Minister the Rt Hon James Callaghan (Labour), delivered at Ruskin College, Oxford, on the mismatch between what was taught in schools and what skills industry was thought to need (see Finn 1982).

3 The proportion of females to males among the new Modern Apprenticeships, launched in 1994, is 37 per cent in England and 24

per cent in Wales. Job segregation is very marked, with most women being in childcare apprenticeships (average weekly pay of £41) and business administration (£45), while young men are found in engineering (where average weekly rates are £88) (EOC).

4 The Department of Employment (DE) was merged with the Department for Education in 1995 to form the Department for Education and Employment (DfEE).

5 In similar vein, Ramazanoglu reports how the group of married women shift-workers she intended to study for her PhD were constructed in her University Department as 'abnormal' and she felt sufficiently discouraged by this response to abandon her studies (Ramazanoglu 1989: 429).

6 In Northern Ireland, responsibility for training lies with the Training and Employment Agency.

7 This chapter draws upon the following projects:

1 Women in Post-compulsory Education and Training in Wales 1994, funded by the Equal Opportunities Commission. See Istance and Rees (1994, 1996). David Istance conducted the statistical work for the study.

2 The Institutional Determinants of Adult Training: The Bridgend Case Study 1988–90. Funded by the Economic and Social Research Council (Grant No. XC1125009). My co-grant holder was Gareth Rees and the research officer was Sarah Fielder. See Rees *et al.* (1991).

I am grateful to my colleagues for their permission to draw upon these studies here.

8 For some young women, pregnancy and motherhood has become an alternative identity to that of student, trainee or employee. This provoked a moral panic about single mothers in the St Mellons housing estate in Cardiff, fuelled in 1994 by the (then) Secretary of State for Wales, John Redwood. The impact of the lack of childcare on women's take-up of training is evidenced by the fact that lone mothers have been identified as a particular group where under-participation is high (Meager and Williams 1994).

9 The figures for undergraduates on which the study was based refers to the period shortly before the Polytechnic of Wales became the University of Glamorgan.

10 General National Vocational Qualifications (GNVQs) were introduced in September 1992 to add a third type of qualification to academic qualifications and NVQs (see Appendix II).

6 SKILL SHORTAGES, WOMEN, AND TRAINING FOR THE NEW INFORMATION TECHNOLOGIES

1 This chapter draws *inter alia* upon two studies I conducted for the EC, one on VET for NITs (Rees 1994b), and the other on skill shortages, women and NITs (1992b), and upon a project on high-level

technology training and women's employment in Wales (Fielder and Rees 1991).

2 Indeed, my mother, along with many other young women from the WRENS (Women's Royal Navy), worked on the Enigma codebreaking project at the crypto-analytical headquarters during the Second World War, using an early model of a computer designed by mathematician Alan Turing to crack secret German, Italian and Japanese armed forces' communication codes (see Hinsley and Stripp 1993).

7 EC COMMUNITY ACTION PROGRAMMES ON EDUCATION AND TRAINING

1 Sources used included interviews with key people responsible for the programmes and others (listed below), analysis of statistics and programme documentation, and internal reports and published reports.

I am particularly grateful to the following for their assistance: Hywel Ceri Jones, Tom O'Dwyer, Frances Smith, David O'Sullivan, Constance Meldrum, Barry Wilson, Judith Grieve, Laura Viquera, Tim Mawson, Rita Vegadacoona (TFHR), Rebecca Franceskides (CREW), Agnes Hubert (DGV Equal Opportunities Unit), Magarida Pinto (DGV Equal Opportunities Unit and later TFHR), Prof. Jacqueline Loufer (consultant to DGV on mainstreaming), Mario Bucci (consultant to TFHR on evaluation of programmes), Anne O'Brien (COMETT TAO), Mieke Grazell, Elizabeth Ogden (ERASMUS TAO), Jack Hogan (EUROTECNET BAT), Jeremy Harrison, Begonia Rodriguez, Adam Ffoulkes Robert (FORCE TAO), Charles Barriere (LINGUA TAO), Betty De Wachter, John Banks (PETRA TAO), Matthew Saier (TEMPUS TAO), John Fells (TEMPUS TAO), members of the Social Dialogue John Rogers (ETUC), Andrew Moore (UNICE), and Claire Molyneux (WITEC UETP COMETT). Isobel Bowler assisted in the data collection phase of the project and the development of the ideas.

Two 'brainstorms' of thirty people from the Task Force, Technical Assistance Offices, DGV Equal Opportunities Unit, CREW/IRIS, CEDEFOP and EURYDICE held on the topic of 'Women and Training' were convened by the Director of the Task Force, before and after the production of the 'Rees Report'. They were extremely timely and fruitful, and allowed for feedback on some of the ideas contained in this report which have been incorporated into this chapter.

Documents analysed include Council Decisions, programme vade-mecums, information brochures, applicants' guidelines, application forms, descriptions, annual reports and evaluation reports, IRIS Bulletins, CREW Reports, and papers presented at the IRIS Fair in October 1992.

Reports consulted included: Banks (1992), Berning (1992), CEC (1991d)(COMETT), Coopers and Lybrand Europe (1992), Coopers and Lybrand, C and L Belmont with the Science Policy Research Unit

(1989), de Jonge and Dillo (1992); de Jonge, Dillo and Mertens (1992), Del Rio Martin *et al.* (n.d.) (PETRA), ECOTEC (1991), ERASMUS Technical Assistance Office (1992), Maiworm *et al.* (1992), PETRA Technical Assistance Office (1989) (1991), Teichler (1991); Teichler *et al.* (1990; 1991a; 1991b; 1992), TFHR (1992).

2   There is a programme-by-programme analysis of programme documentation in Appendix II of Rees (1995b)

8   THE EUROPEAN SOCIAL FUND AND LEONARDO DA VINCI

1   All three White Papers are discussed in some detail in Chapter 9.

2   The Programmes were renamed *Transition from Education to Adult Life*. In the context of high youth unemployment rates, the name change was introduced because it was thought that young people were at least highly likely to become adults even if they were not necessarily to be afforded an opportunity to engage in working life. Coincidentally, some twenty years later, I find my young sons also adopt this strategy. When asked what they would like to be when they grow up, they both invariably reply 'a man'.

3   See Callender (1991) for an account of the UK study.

4   For an assessment of the lessons which can be drawn from the experience of the IRIS network in Germany, see Wilpert (1996), and in France, see Beaumelou and Mora-Canzini (1996).

5   The author is the coordinator of Project Mosaic. The research partners are Esther Appelo of Dreikant (Netherlands), Franca Bimbi, University of Padua (Italy), Agneta Stark, University of Stockholm (Sweden), Tom Casey of Circa (Ireland) and Binna Kandola of Pearn Kandola (UK).

9   COMPETITIVENESS, SOCIAL EXCLUSION AND THE LEARNING SOCIETY

1   Earlier versions of this chapter were presented at the Wales–Baden Wurttemberg Colloquium organised by the University of Tübingen in 1996, and at the *International Planning Studies* workshop on social exclusion held at the University of Wales Cardiff in 1997. I am grateful to colleagues for helpful comments.

2   Indeed, I worked as a research fellow on the Upper Afan Community Development Project in South Wales in the early 1970s as part of the Home Office's Combat Poverty programme. The Upper Afan Valley is an ex-mining community.

3   In preparing my critique of the chapter on education and training in the White Paper (Rees 1995a), I benefited considerably from debates with my six academic colleagues and from staff from the Equal Opportunities Unit. The impact of DGV's Equal Opportunities Unit can also be seen in the 1995 edition of the annual publication *Employment in Europe* (EC 1995a) where Jill Rubery and others were

commissioned to 'gender-proof' the draft document, ensuring that, unlike in previous editions, gender differences were highlighted rather than ignored.

4 Eurostat defines poverty as a situation in which people live in households where the expenditure per equivalent adult is less than half the national average.

10 MAINSTREAMING EQUALITY

1 I am grateful to the EOC for this information.

APPENDIX III

1 ECOSOC Information Report on Vocational Training, 'The promotion of vocational qualifications – an instrument for the economic and social development of the European Community', CES 587/92 final.

It is widely agreed that high-quality skills are of strategic importance for EC integration. They boost business productivity and competitiveness, improve workers' living and working conditions and enhance their employment prospects.

2 Joint Opinion on Ways of Facilitating the Broadest Possible Effective Access to Training Opportunities, 20 December 1991, preamble 4.

3 Between 1985 and 1990, two-thirds of new jobs created in the Community were taken by women.

4 Gender segregation persists in all EC countries and women are concentrated in fewer economic sectors than men.

5 These views are supported by the OECD, whose 1992 'Women and Structural change' recorded: 'The solution to economic problems depends on enhancing women's economic role. Women are a key resource that is currently under-utilised both quantitatively and qualitatively.'

Similarly, the EC Standing Committee on Employment (1991) recognises the important role women will play in economic and social cohesion: 'Better qualitative and quantitative integration of women into both long term employment and posts involving responsibility is an important factor for the Community's economic and social cohesion'.

6 1 Joint Opinion on Education and Training (19 June 1990)
  2 Joint Opinion on the Transition from School to Adult and Working Life (5 April 1991)
  3 Joint Opinion on Ways of Facilitating the Broadest Possible Effective Access to Training Opportunities (20 December 1991)
  4 Joint Opinion on Vocational Qualifications and Certification (13 October 1992).

Bibliography

Aaron, J. and Walby, S. (eds) (1991) *Out of the Margins: Women's Studies in the Nineties* Brighton: Falmer.

Acker, S. (1992) 'Critical Introduction: Travel and Travail' in J. Gaskell *School, Work and Gender* Milton Keynes: Open University Press.

Allen, I. (1988) *Any Room at the Top? A Study of Doctors and their Careers* London: Policy Studies Institute.

Arber, S. and Ginn, J. (1991) *Gender and Later Life: a sociological analysis of resources and constraints* London: Sage.

Archer, C. and Butler, F. (1996) *The European Union* (second edition) London: Sage.

Arnot, M., David, M. and Weiner, G. (1996) *Educational Reforms and Gender Equality in Schools* Manchester: Equal Opportunities Commission.

Association of University Teachers (1992) 'Sex Discrimination in Universities: report of an academic pay audit carried out by the AUT Research Department' London: AUT.

Atkinson, P. and Delamont, S. (1990) 'Professions and powerlessness: female marginality in the learned occupations' *Sociological Review* Vol. 38, No. 1, pp. 90–110.

Awbery, G. (1997) *The Sex Discrimination Act and the Use of Welsh in the Workplace* Manchester: Equal Opportunities Commission.

Bagihole, B. (1993) 'How to keep a good woman down: an investigation into the role of institutional factors in the process of discrimination against women academics' *British Journal of Sociology of Education* Vol. 14, No. 3, pp. 261–71.

Banks, J. (1992) 'The European Network of Training Partnerships: The First (1988) Projects and their Transnational Partnerships' Annex A, Brussels: PETRA Technical Assistance Office.

Beaumelou, F. and Mora-Canzini, F. (1996) *L'Europe et la Formation des Femmes* Paris: Racine.

Beccalli, B. (1984) 'Italy' in A. H. Cooke, V. R. Lorwin and A. K. Daniels (eds) *Women and Trade Unions in Eleven Industrialised Countries* Philadelphia: Temple University Press.

Beccalli, B. and Salvati, M. (1995) 'Gender, Employment and Working Time: A Long-run View' in European Commission *Equal Opportunities for Women and Men: Follow-up to the White Paper on Growth, Competitiveness and Employment* Report to the European Commission's Task Force (Directorate-General V) Brussels: DGV European Commission V/5538/95-EN.

Beechey, V. (1987) *Unequal Work* London: Verso.

Berghman, J. (1995) 'Social exclusion in Europe: policy context and analytical framework' in G. Room (ed.) *The Measurement and Analysis of Social Exclusion* Bristol: Policy Press.

Berning, E. (1992) *Accommodation of ERASMUS-students in the Member States of the European Community* Brussels: Commission of the European Communities.

Bernstein, B. (1971) *Class, Codes and Control* Vol. 1, London: Paladin.

Birchard, M. (1997) 'Mainstreaming: DfEE Permanent Secretary outlines his Department's approach to mainstreaming' in Department for Education and Employment/EOC (1997) *Fair Play National Newsletter No. 6*, London: DfEE/EOC, p. 9.

Blackburn, R. M., Jarman, J. and Siltanen, J. (1993) 'The Analysis of Occupational Gender Segregation over Time and Place: Considerations of Measurement and Some New Evidence' *Work, Employment and Society* Vol. 7, No. 3. pp. 335–62.

—— (1994a) 'A Reply to Lampard' *Work, Employment and Society*, Vol. 8, No. 3, pp. 413–19.

—— (1994b) 'A Reply to Watts' *Work, Employment and Society*, Vol. 8, No. 3, pp. 433–8.

Blackley, S. (1994) *Managing Innovative and Transnational Training Projects: A Guide to Good Practice and a complete Directory of British EUROFORM projects* Leeds: Industrial Common Ownership Movement.

Blackley, S., Goddard, M. and Seymour, H. (1995) *Innovative and Transnational Projects: a guide for organisations running projects supported by the European Structural Funds, Community Action Programmes, or other European Commission sources* Leeds: Industrial Common Ownership Movement.

Boddendijk, F. R. (1991) 'The long way to equal opportunities for women and men' in Commission of the European Communities *Equal Opportunities for Women and Men: Social Europe Supplement 3/91* Directorate General for Employment, Industrial Relations and Social Affairs, Luxembourg: Office for Official Publications of the European Communities, pp. 94–7.

Boddy, M. (1995) *TECs and Racial Equality: training and work experience for ethnic minorities* Bristol: University of Bristol, SAUS Publications.

Brah, A. (1991) 'Questions of Difference and International Feminism' in J. Aaron and S. Walby (eds) *Out of the Margins* London: Falmer.

Brannen, J. and Moss, P. (1991) *Managing Mothers – Dual Earner Households* London: Unwin Hyman.

Breakthrough (1994) 'European Network for Women's Local Employment Initiatives' *Dossier 6* Thessaloniki: LEI European Coordination, Breakthrough.

Breakwell, G. (1985) *The Quiet Rebel: Women at Work in a Man's World* London: Century Publishing.

Breugal, I. and Hegewisch, A. (1994) 'Flexibilisation and part-time work in Europe' in P. Brown and R. Crompton (eds) *Economic Restructuring and Social Exclusion* London: UCL Press.

Breugal, I. and Perrons, D. (1995) 'Where do the costs of unequal treatment for women fall? An analysis of the incidence of the costs of unequal pay and sex discrimination in the UK' in J. Humphries and J. Rubery (eds) *The Economics of Equal Opportunities* Manchester: Equal Opportunities Commission.

Brine, J. (1992) 'The European Social Fund and the vocational training of unemployed women: questions of gendering and regendering' *Gender and Education* Vol. 4, No. 1–2, pp. 149–62.

—— (1995a) 'Equal Opportunities and the European Social Fund: discourse and practice' *Gender and Education* Vol. 7, No. 1, pp. 9–22.

—— (1995b) 'Educational and vocational policy and the construction of the European Union' *International Studies in Sociology of Education* Vol. 5, No. 2, pp. 145–63.

Brown, P. (1994) 'Education, Training and Economic Change' *Work Employment and Society* Vol. 8, No. 4, pp. 607–21.

Brown, P. and Crompton, R. (eds) (1994) *Economic Restructuring and Social Exclusion* London: UCL Press.

Bucci, M. (1991) *Report on the Access of Young People to Community Programmes in the Field of Education and Training* Internal Report, EC Task Force Human Resources, Education, Training and Youth.

Business in the Community (1992) *Opportunity 2000 annual report* London: Business in the Community.

—— (1993) *Opportunity 2000 annual report* London: Business in the Community.

Bynner, J. and Fogelman, K. (1993) 'Making the Grade: Education and Training Experiences' in E. Ferri (ed.) *Life at 33: The Fifth Follow-up of the National Child Development Study* London: National Children's Bureau.

Callender, C. (1991) *Women's Participation in Actions Co-financed by the European Social Fund* Final Report Brighton: Institute of Manpower Studies.

—— (1994) *Running Training Schemes for Women: A Good Practice Guide and Directory of NOW Projects 1990–1994* London: Women's Training Network and Industrial Common Ownership Movement.

Campanelli, P., Thomas, R., Channell, J., McAulay, L. and Renouf, A. (1994) 'Training: an exploration of the word and the concept with an analysis of the implications for survey design' *Research Series No. 30* London: Employment Department.

Carter, S. and Cannon, T. (1988) 'Female entrepreneurs: a study of female business owners, their motivations, experiences and strategies for success' *Research Paper No. 65*, London: Employment Department.

Cary, M. (1995) *Women in Non-traditional Employment in Northern Ireland* Unpublished PhD thesis, Queen's University Belfast.

Castelberg-Koulma, M. (1991) 'Greek Women and Tourism: Women's co-operatives as an alternative form of organization' in N. Redclift and M. Thea Sinclair (eds) *Working Women: International Perspectives on Labour and Gender Ideology* London: Routledge.

CEEP, ETUC and UNICE (1995) *Women and Training in Europe: 50 projects which challenge our traditions* A Compendium of Good Practice, published at the initiative of the European Social Dialogue, Brussels: DGXXII European Commission.

Central Statistical Office (1993) *Regional Trends 28, 1993 Edition* London: HMSO.

—— (1995) *Regional Trends 30, 1995 Edition* London: HMSO.

Chancellor of the Duchy of Lancaster (1993) *Realising our Potential: A Strategy for Science, Engineering and Technology* London: HMSO Cmnd 2250.

Christiansen, D. (1992) *Female Participation in the Training Programmes of the TFHR* Paper presented to the European Commission/Social Dialogue seminar on women, training and equal opportunities, held in Madrid, February 1992.

Christie, I., Northcott, J. and Walling, A. (1990) *Employment Effects of New Technology in Manufacturing* London: Policy Studies Institute.

Clarke, K. (1991) 'Women and Training: A Review' *Equal Opportunities Research Discussion Series No. 1* Manchester: Equal Opportunities Commission.

Coats, M. (1994) *Women's Education* Buckingham: Open University Press.

Cockburn, C. (1983) *Brothers: Male Dominance and Technological Change* London: Pluto Press.

—— (1985) *Machinery of Dominance: Women, Men and Technical Know-how* London: Pluto.

—— (1986) 'Women and New Technology: Opportunity is Not Enough' in K. Purcell, S. Woods, A. Waton and S. Allen (eds) *The Changing Experience of Employment: Restructuring and Recession* London: Macmillan.

—— (1987) *Two Track Training: Sex Inequalities and the Youth Training Scheme* London: Macmillan.

—— (1989) 'EO: the short and the long agenda' *Industrial Relations Journal* Vol. 20, No. 3, pp. 213–25.

—— (1991) *In the Way of Women: Men's Resistance to Sex Equality in Organisations* London: Macmillan.

Cockburn, C. and Ormrod, S. (1993) *Gender and Technology in the Making* London: Sage.

Coe, T. (1992) *The Key to the Men's Club: opening the doors to women in management* London: Institute of Management.

Cohen, B. (1990) *Caring for Children: The 1990 Report* London: Family Policy Studies.

Collin, F. (1992) *Le Sexe des Sciences, les Femmes en Plus Série: Science et Société* No. 6, Editions, Paris: Autrement.

Collins, H. (1992) *The Equal Opportunities Handbook* Oxford: Blackwell.

Collinson, D., Knights, D. and Collinson, M. (1990) *Managing to Discriminate* London: Routledge.

Commission for Racial Equality (1991) *TECs and Racial Equality: An*

Agenda for Equal Opportunities London: Commission for Racial Equality.

—— (1992) *TECs and Racial Equality: Equal Access to Jobs and Training – Handbook for TECs and LECs on positive action, targeted training and customised training* London: Commission for Racial Equality.

Commission of the European Communities (1987a) *Non-salaried Working Women in Europe: Women Running their own Businesses or Working Independently – Women Involved in their Husband's Professional Activity* Brussels: Commission of the European Communities.

—— (1987b) 'Commission Recommendation of 24 November 1987 on vocational training for women' *Official Journal of the European Communities* No. 1 342/35, 4 December 1987.

—— (1989) *Guide to the European Community Programme in the Fields of Education, Training and Youth* EC Task Force Human Resources, Education, Training and Youth.

—— (1990) *Equal Opportunities for Women and Men: The Third Medium Term Community Action Programme 1991–1995* Brussels CEC COM(90)449 (final).

—— (1991a) *Equal Opportunities for Women and Men: The Third Medium Term Community Action Programme 1991–1995* Women of Europe Supplements No. 34, Commission of the European Communities, Directorate-General Audio-visual, Information, Communication, Culture; Women's Information Service.

—— (1991b) *Equal Opportunities for Women and Men* Social Europe 3/91, Directorate-General for Employment, Industrial Relations and Social Affairs, Luxembourg: Office for Official Publications of the European Communities.

—— (1991c) *Synopsis of the Activities of the Task Force Human Resources, Education, Training and Youth of the Commission of the European Communities during 1989/1990* Brussels: Commission of the European Communities.

—— (1991d) *COMETT I: Final Report of the Commission (1986–1990)* Brussels: CEC Sec(91)1016 (final).

—— (1992) *The Position of Women on the Labour Market: Trends and Developments in the Twelve Member States of the European Community 1983–1990* Brussels: Commission of the European Communities, Directorate General Audio-visual, Information, Communication, Culture; Women's Information Service.

—— (1992a) *Report on the Activities of the Commission of the European Communities in the Field of Education, Training and Youth During 1990* (presented by the Commission) SEC(91) 2409 final 24th January, Brussels: Commission of the European Communities.

—— (1992b) 'Participation in the Evaluation of the Comett Programme: Notice of Invitation to Tender' (TFHR/03/92) (92/C 143/04) *Official Journal of the European Communities*, 5 June 1992.

—— (1992c) 'Evaluation of the COMETT Programme Tender Document (in relation to Call for Tender)' (TFHR/03/92) CC/10/5 JCS/6/5 Brussels: Commission of the European Communities.

—— (1993a) *Women and Training: Experience of the Community Initiative*

NOW (New Opportunities for Women) Report prepared for the Social Dialogue at Community level and its *ad hoc* working group on Education and Training in the context of a discussion on women and training. Brussels: Commission of the European Communities, DGV European Social Fund V/D/1.

—— (1993b) *EC Education and Training Programmes 1986–1992. Results and Achievements: An Overview* Luxembourg: Office for Official Publications of the European Communities COM(93) 151 (final).

—— (1993c) *Guide to the European Community Programmes in the Fields of Education, Training and Youth* Brussels: Commission of the European Communities, Task Force Human Resources, Education, Training and Youth.

—— (1993d) *Skills for a Competitive Europe: A Human Resource Outlook for the 1990s* 2nd edn, Brussels: DGXXII, Commission of the European Communities.

—— (1993e) *European Social Policy: Options for the Future*, Green Paper, DGV, Luxembourg: Office for Official Publications of the European Communities.

—— (1993f) *Guidelines for Community Action in the Field of Education and Training* (the 'Ruberti Guidelines'), COM(93) 183 final, Brussels: Commission of the European Communities.

—— (1995a) *Proposal for a Council Decision on the Fourth Medium Term Action Programme on Equal Opportunities for Women and Men (1996–2000)* COM(95) 381 (final) Brussels: Commission of the European Communities.

—— (1995b) '9th May, Europe Day' *Women of Europe No. 51* DGX Brussels: Commission of the European Communities .

—— (1996) *Incorporating Equal Opportunities for Women and Men into all Community Policies and Activities*, Communication from the Commission, COM(96) 67 (final), Luxembourg: Office for Official Publications of the European Communities.

Commission of the European Communities and Social Dialogue (1993) *Joint Opinion on Women and Training* SEC(93) 1977 Brussels: Commission of the European Communities.

Commission on Social Justice (1994) *Social Justice: Strategies for National Renewal*, The Report of the Commission on Social Justice, London: Vintage.

Confederation of British Industry (1989) *Towards a Skills Revolution* Report of the Vocational Education and Training Task Force, London: CBI.

Cooke, P. (1996) 'Regions in a Global Market: The Experiences of Wales and Baden-Wurttemburg', paper delivered to the 1996 Wales–Baden-Wurttemburg Colloquium, University of Tübingen.

Coopers and Lybrand, C. and L. Belmont, with the Science Policy Research Unit, University of Sussex (1989) *Evaluation of the COMETT Programme* Brussels: Commission of the European Communities, Task Force Human Resources, Education, Training and Youth.

Coopers and Lybrand Europe (1992) *Evaluation of the TEMPUS Programme* Brussels: Coopers and Lybrand Europe.

Cormack, R. J. and Osborne, R. D. (eds) (1991) *Discrimination and Public Policy in Northern Ireland* Oxford: Clarendon Press.

—— (1993) *Religion, Education and Employment: Aspects of Equal Opportunity in Northern Ireland* Belfast: Appletree Press.

Council of the European Community and Commission of the European Communities (1992) *Treaty on European Union* (The 'Maastricht Treaty') Brussels: Commission of the European Communities.

Cox, S. (1993) 'Equal Opportunities' in M. Gold (ed.) *The Social Dimension: Employment Policy in the European Community* London: Macmillan.

Coyle, A. (1995) *Women and Organisational Change* Research Discussion Series No. 14, Manchester: Equal Opportunities Commission.

Cringely, R. X. (1992) *Accidental Empires – how the boys of Silicon Valley make their millions, battle foreign competition, and still can't get a date* Harmondsworth: Penguin.

Crompton, R. (1987) 'Gender, Status and Professionalism' *Sociology* Vol. 21, No. 3, pp. 413–28.

Crompton, R. and Brown, P. (1994) 'Introduction' in P. Brown and R. Crompton (eds) *Economic Restructuring and Social Exclusion* London: UCL Press.

Crompton, R. and Sanderson, K. (1990a) *Gendered Jobs and Social Change* London: Unwin Hyman.

—— (1990b) 'Credentials and Careers' in G. Payne and P. Abbott (eds) *The Social Mobility of Women* Basingstoke: Falmer Press.

Cunningham, S. (1992) 'The development of equal opportunities theory and practice in the European Community' *Policy and Politics* Vol. 20, No. 3, pp. 177–89.

Curran, C. (1995) *The potential cost-effectiveness of tertiary open and distance learning* Luxembourg: Office for Official Publications of the European Communities.

Daly, M. (1979) *Gyn Ecology* London: The Women's Press.

David, M. (1983) 'Sex education and social policy: a new moral economy?' in S. Walker and L. Barton (eds) *Gender, Class and Education* London: Falmer.

Davidson, M. J. and Cooper, C. L. (eds) (1987) *Women and Information Technology* London: Wiley.

de Bruijn, J. (1995) 'Equal Opportunities and New Requirements for New Jobs' in European Commission *Equal Opportunities for Women and Men: Follow-up to the White Paper on Growth, Competitiveness and Employment* Report to the European Commission's Task Force (DGV) Brussels: DGV European Commission V/5538/95-EN.

de Jonge, J. F. M. and Dillo, I. G. (1992) *Student Mobility in Higher Education in the European Community, Vol. I. (Synthesis Report)* Brussels: Commission of the European Communities.

de Jonge, J. F. M., Dillo, I. G. and Mertens, R. M. (1992) *Student Mobility in Higher Education in the European Community, Vol. II* Brussels: Commission of the European Communities.

Deem, R. (ed.) (1984) *Co-education Reconsidered* Milton Keynes: Open University Press.

Degimbe, J. (1991) 'Foreword' in Commission of the European Communities *Equal Opportunities for Women and Men: Social Europe Supplement 3/91* Directorate General for Employment Industrial Relations and Social Affairs, Luxembourg: Office for Official Publications of the European Communities.

Delamont, S. (1994) *Appetites and Identities: An Introduction to the Social Anthropology of Western Europe* London: Routledge.

Del Rio Martin, E., Fourmy, C., Gathier, P., Nacken, W. and Douglas, H. (n. d.) *Evaluation of the Youth Initiative Projects of the PETRA Programme* Madrid: Centro de Información, Gestión y Promoción del Empleo Juvenil.

Department for Education (1993) *Statistical Bulletin on Women in Post-compulsory Education* Issue 26/93 December, London: Department for Education.

Department for Education and Employment/EOC (1997) *Fair Play National Newsletter No. 6*, London: DfEE/EOC.

Department for Education and Employment, Scottish Office and Welsh Office (1995) *Lifetime Learning: A Consultation Document* Sheffield: DfEE.

Deroure, F. (1990) *Accompanying Measures in Women's Training: Vocational Training for Women* Brussels: DGV, Commission of the European Communities.

—— (1992) *Professional Mobility in Europe: Family Aspects and Business Practices* Brussels: DGV, Commission of the European Communities.

—— (1993) *La Formation Professionelle des Femmes dans la Communauté* Brussels: Report to DGV, Commission of the European Communities.

Dex, S. (1988) *Women's Attitudes to Work* London: Macmillan.

Dick, A. and Faulstich-Wieland, H. (1988) 'Der hessiche Modellversuch "Madchenbildung und Neue Technolgien"' in *LOG IN* 8, No. 1.

Dinan, D. (1994) *Ever Closer Union? An Introduction to the European Community* Basingstoke: Macmillan.

Doogan, K. (in press) 'The impact of European integration on labour market institutions' *International Planning Studies*.

Ducatel, K. (ed.) (1994) *Employment and Technical Change in Europe: Work Organisation, Skills and Training* Cheltenham: Edward Elgar.

Ducatel, K. and Miles, I. (1990) *New Information Technologies and Working Conditions in the European Communities* Employment and Training Perspectives in the New Information Technologies in the European Community Project, Report to the EC Task Force Human Resources, Education, Training and Youth, Manchester: University of Manchester; Brighton: Science Policy Research Unit.

—— (1994) *New Information Technologies and Working Conditions in the European Communities* Report to EC Task Force Human Resources, Education Training and Youth, Employment and Training Perspectives in the New Information Technologies in the European Community Project, Manchester: University of Manchester; and Brighton: Science Policy Research Unit.

Duncan, S. (1996) 'Obstacles to a Successful Equal Opportunities Policy in the European Union' *European Journal of Women's Studies*, Vol. 3, No. 4, pp. 399–422.

Durndell, A. and Thomson, K. (1997) 'Gender and Computing: A decade of change?' *Computers and Education* Vol. 28, No. 1, pp. 1–9.

ECOTEC (1991) *Evaluation of COMETT*, Report to the EC Task Force Human Resources, Education, Training and Youth.

Employment Department (1993) *Training Statistics 1993* London: HMSO.

—— (1995) *Training Statistics 1995* London: HMSO.

Equal Opportunities Commission (1993) *Formal Investigation into the Publicly-funded Vocational Training System in England and Wales* Manchester: Equal Opportunities Commission.

—— (1996a) *Challenging Inequalities between Women and Men: twenty years of progress 1976–96* Manchester: Equal Opportunities Commission.

—— (1996b) *Briefing on Mainstreaming* Manchester: Equal Opportunities Commission.

ERASMUS Technical Assistance Office (1992) 'Female participation in the ERASMUS Programme 1987/88–1990/91', Annex to the briefing on ERASMUS and Equal Opportunities, Brussels: ERASMUS Technical Assistance Office.

Eriksson, I. V., Kitchenham, B. and Tijdens, K. G. (eds) (1991) *Women, Work and Computerization: Understanding and Overcoming Bias in Work and Education* Amsterdam: North-Holland.

Escott, K. and Whitfield, D. (1995) *The Gender Impact of CCT in Local Government* Research Discussion Series No. 12, Manchester: Equal Opportunities Commission.

Essex, S., Callender, C., Rees, T. and Winckler, V. (1986) *New Styles of Training for Women: An Evaluation of the South Glamorgan Women's Workshop* Manchester: Equal Opportunities Commission.

European Commission (1994a) *Growth, Competitiveness, Employment: The Challenges and Ways Forward into the 21st Century* White Paper. Bulletin of the Commission of the European Communities Supplement 6/93 Luxembourg: Office for Official Publications of the European Communities.

—— (1994b) *European Social Policy: A Way Forward for The Union* Luxembourg: Office for Official Publications of the European Communities.

—— (1994c) *Women at the European Commission from 1984 to 1994* Brussels/Luxembourg: Commission of the European Communities.

—— (1994d) *Higher Education in the European Union: Facts and Figures over a Decade* Luxembourg: Office for Official Publications of the European Commission.

—— (1994e) *Contributions to the Preparatory Work for the White Paper on European Social Policy* DGV Social Europe 2/94, Luxembourg: Office for Official Publications of the European Communities.

—— (1995a) *Employment in Europe 1995* Luxembourg: Office for Official Publications of the European Communities.

—— (1995b) *Two Years of Social Policy: July 1993–June 1995*, Social

Europe 3/94, Luxembourg: Office for Official Publications of the European Communities.

—— (1995c) *Eurotecnet: action programme for the promotion of innovation in vocational training resulting from technological change: compendium of innovation* DGXXII, Luxembourg: Office for Official Publications of the European Communities.

—— (1995d) *Equal Opportunities for Women and Men: Follow-up to the White Paper on Growth, Competitiveness and Employment* Report to the European Commission's Task Force (DGV), Brussels: DGV, European Commission V/5538/95-EN.

—— (1996a) *Fourth Medium-Term Community Action Programme on EO for Men and Women (1996–2000)* Brussels: DGV, European Commission V/231b/96-EN.

—— (1996b) *Teaching and Learning: Towards the Learning Society* Luxembourg: Office for Official Publications of the European Communities.

—— (1996c) 'Court of Justice: Positive discrimination challenged' *Women of Europe Newsletter*, No. 57, Brussels: DGX, European Commission.

—— (1996d) *LEONARDO DA VINCI. Innovative Training for Europe: Products Catalogue* Brussels: DGXXII, European Commission.

—— (1996e) *LEONARDO DA VINCI. Innovative Training for Europe: Proceedings of the Products Fair, 18, 19, 20 April 1996* Brussels: DGXXII, European Commission.

—— (1997) *Annual Report from the Commission: Equal Opportunities for Women and Men in the European Union* COM(96) 650 (final), Luxembourg: Office for Official Publications of the European Communities.

European Foundation for the Improvement of Living and Working Conditions (1994) *Families, Labour Markets and Gender Roles* Dublin: EFILWC.

Eurostat (1992) *Women in the European Community* Luxembourg: Office for Official Publications of the European Commission.

—— (1995a) *Women and Men in the European Union* Luxembourg: Office for Official Publications of the Commission of the European Communities.

—— (1995b) *Eurostat Key Figures: Bulletin of Economic Trends in Europe* 07/95, Luxembourg: Office for Official Publications of the Commission of the European Communities.

—— (1996) *Social Portrait of Europe* Luxembourg: Office for Official Publications of the Commission of the European Communities.

Fagnani, J. (1996) 'Family Policies and Working Mothers: a comparison of France and Germany' in M. D. García-Ramon and J. Monk (eds) *Women of the European Union: the politics of work and daily life* London: Routledge.

Felstead, A. (1995) 'The Gender Implications of Creating a Training Market: Alleviating or Reinforcing Inequality of Access?' in J. Humphries and J. Rubery (eds) *The Economics of Equal Opportunities* Manchester: Equal Opportunities Commission.

—— (1996) 'Identifying Gender Inequalities in the Distribution of

Vocational Qualifications in the UK' *Gender, Work and Organisation* Vol. 3, No. 1, pp. 38–50.

Field, J. (1995) *Spicers European Union Briefings: Employment Policy* London: Catermill Publishing.

Fielder, S. and Rees, T. (1991) *High Level Information Technology Training and Women's Employment* Cardiff: Social Research Unit, University of Wales Cardiff.

Finch, J. (1983) *Married to the Job* London: George Allen and Unwin.

Finn, D. (1982) 'Whose needs? Schooling and the needs of industry' in T. Rees and P. Atkinson (eds) *Youth Unemployment and State Intervention* London: Routledge and Kegan Paul.

Flynn, P. (1996) 'Fourth Community Action Programme for Women and Men (1996–2000): Mechanisms for Mainstreaming' Speech delivered at the EC's *Mechanisms for Mainstreaming* conference during the Irish Presidency, Dublin.

Fogarty, M., Allen, I. and Walters, P. (1981) *Women in Top Jobs 1968–79* London: Heinemann/Policy Studies Institute.

Foucault, M. (1980) *Power-knowledge: selected interview and other writings 1972–1977* New York: Pantheon.

Franceskides, R. and de Troy, C. (eds) (1994) *A Wider Vision: Reflections of Women's Training* Brussels: IRIS European Coordination.

Freeman, C. and Soete, L. (1990) *Macro-Economic and Sectoral Analysis of Future Employment and Training Perspectives in the New Information Technologies in the European Community* Executive Summary, Synthesis Report and Policy Conclusions and Recommendations, Reports to the Task Force Human Resources, Education Training and Youth, Employment and Training Perspectives in the New Information Technologies in the European Community Project.

—— (1991) *Macro-Economic and Sectoral Analysis of Future Employment and Training Perspectives in the New Information Technologies in the European Community* Report to the Task Force Human Resources, Education, Training and Youth.

Gallie, D. (1991) 'Patterns of Skill Change: Upskilling, Deskilling or the Polarization of Skills' *Work Employment and Society* Vol. 5, No. 3, pp. 319–51.

Garland, P. (1994) 'Educating Rhian: Experiences of mature women students' in J. Aaron, T. Rees, S. Betts and M. Vincentelli (eds) *Our Sisters' Land: The Changing Identities of Women in Wales* Cardiff: University of Wales Press.

Gaskell, J. (1986) 'Conceptions of skill and the work of women: some historical and political issues' in R. Hamilton and M. Barrett (eds) *The Politics of Diversity* London: Verso.

Gershuny, J., Anderson, M. and Bechhofer, F. (1994) (eds) *The Social and Political Economy of the Household* Oxford: Oxford University Press.

Gershuny, J., Miles, I., Jones, S., Mullings, C., Thomas, G. and Wyatt, S. (1986) 'Time Budgets: Preliminary Analyses of a National Survey' *Quarterly Journal of Social Affairs* Vol. 2, No. 1, pp. 13–39.

Ginn, J. and Arber, S. (1996) 'Patterns of Employment, Gender and

Pensions: The effect of work history on older women's non-state pension' *Work Employment and Society* Vol. 10, No. 3, pp. 469–90.

Green, F. and Ashton, D. G. (1989) 'Skill Shortage and Skill Deficiency: A Critique' *Work Employment and Society* Vol. 6, No. 2, pp. 287–301.

Gregory, J. (1987) *Sex, Race and the Law: Legislating for Equality* London: Sage.

—— (1992) 'Equal Value/Comparable Worth: National Statute and Case Law in Britain and the USA' in P. Kahn and S. Meehan (eds) *Equal Value/Comparable Worth in the UK and USA* Basingstoke: Macmillan.

Hakim, C. (1989) 'New recruits to self-employment in the 1980s' *Employment Gazette* Vol. 97, No. 6, pp. 286–97.

—— (1993) 'The Myth of Rising Female Employment' *Work Employment and Society* Vol. 7, No. 1, pp. 97–120.

Halsey, A. H. (1977) 'Towards meritocracy' in J. Harabel and A. H. Halsey (eds) *Power and Ideology in Education* New York: Oxford University Press.

Hammond, V. (1992) 'Opportunity 2000: A culture change approach to equal opportunities' *Women in Management Review* Vol. 7, No. 7, pp. 3–10.

Hammond, V. and Holten, V. (1991) 'A Balanced Workforce? Achieving cultural change for women: a comparative study', Research project sponsored by the Women's Economic Development Target Team, Business in the Community for Opportunity 2000, Ashridge: Ashridge Management Centre.

Hansard Society Commission on Women at the Top (1990) *Report of the Hansard Society Commission on Women at the Top* London: The Hansard Society.

Hardill, I. and Green, A. (1990) *An Examination of Women Returners in Benwell and South Gosforth* Newcastle: University of Newcastle upon Tyne, Centre for Urban and Regional Studies.

Harrison, J. (1996) 'Community Initiatives' Presentation at a seminar on ADAPT, held at the School for Policy Studies, University of Bristol.

Healy, G. and Kraithman, D. (1989) *Women Returners in the North Hertfordshire Labour Market* Report for the Training Agency, Hertford: Hatfield Polytechnic, Local Economy Research Unit.

Heward, C. M. (1994) 'Academic Snakes and Merit Ladders: reconceptualising the glass ceiling' *Gender and Education* Vol. 6, No. 3, pp. 249–62.

High Level Group of Experts (1996) *Building the European Information Society for Us All: First Reflections of the High Level Group of Experts* Brussels: DGV, European Commission.

Hinsley, F. H. and Stripp, A. (eds) (1993) *Codebreakers: The Inside Story of Bletchley Park* Oxford: Oxford University Press.

Hirdmann, Y. (1990) *Att Lägga Livet till Rätta; studier i svensk folkhemspolitik* Stockholm: Carlsson.

Hobson, B. (1997) 'Cross National Dialogues and the Emergence of New Waves of Comparative Gender Research in Sweden' in E. Hemlin (ed.) *Det har ända hänt fantastiskt mycket. Vad har jämställdhetsforskningen uppnått* (Gender Equality in Research and Higher Education in

Sweden), Stockholm: Riksbankens Jubileumsfond i samarbete met Gidlunds Förlag.

Holland, J. (1988) 'Girls and Occupational Choice: in search of meanings' in A. Pollard, J. Purvis and G. Walford (eds) *Education, Training and the New Vocationalism* Milton Keynes: Open University Press.

Horrell, S., Rubery, J. and Burchell, B. (1989) 'Unequal Jobs or Unequal Pay?' *Industrial Relations Journal* Vol. 20, No. 3, pp. 176–91.

—— (1990) 'Gender and Skills' *Work Employment and Society* Vol. 4, No. 2, pp. 176–216.

Hoskyns, C. (1988) ' "Give us equal pay and we'll open our own doors" – a study of the impact in the Federal Republic of Germany and the Republic of Ireland of the European Community's policy on women's rights' in M. Buckley and M. Anderson (eds) *Women, Equality and Europe* Basingstoke: Macmillan.

—— (1992) 'The European Community's Policy on Women in the Context of 1992' *Women's Studies International Forum* Vol. 15, No. 1, pp. 21–8.

—— (1996) *Integrating Gender: Women, Law and Politics in the European Union* London: Verso.

Hoskyns, C. and Luckhaus, L. (1989) 'The EC Directive on Equal Treatment in Social Security' *Policy and Politics* Vol. 17, No. 4, pp. 321–36.

Humm, M. (1989) *The Dictionary of Feminist Theory* Hemel Hempstead: Harvester Wheatsheaf.

Humphries, J. and Rubery, J. (eds) (1995) *The Economics of Equal Opportunities* Manchester: Equal Opportunities Commission.

Hunt, D. (1993) *Helper Spouse: European Enterprise and Training Policy* Report to DGV, Commission of the European Communities, Cork: Centre for Vocational Training and Sectoral Analysis, University College Cork.

Hutson, S. and Liddiard, M. (1994) *Youth Homelessness: The Construction of a Social Issue* London: Macmillan.

Hutton, W. (1995) *The State We're In* London: Cape.

Huws, U. (1995) *Teleworking, Social Europe Supplement 3/95* Luxembourg: Office for Official Publications of the European Communities.

IRDAC (1991) *Skill Shortages in Europe: IRDAC Opinion* Brussels: Industrial Research and Development Advisory Committee of the Commission of the European Communities.

IRIS (1993) *IRIS Network Directory 1993* Brussels: Centre for Research on Women (CREW).

—— (n.d.) *Evaluation: An IRIS Network report on evaluation techniques, practices and innovation in women's training* Brussels: Centre for Research on Women (CREW).

IRIS/CREW (n.d.) *Submission for Social Policy Green Paper: An Insight into Women's Training by the IRIS Office/CREW* Brussels: Centre for Research on Women (CREW).

Istance, D. and Rees, T. (1994) *Women in Post Compulsory Education and Training in Wales* Research Discussion Series No. 8, Manchester: Equal Opportunities Commission.

—— (1996) 'Escaping the Low Wage/Low Skill Syndrome in Wales: The

Case for Investing in Women's Skills' *British Journal of Education and Work*, Vol. 9, No. 1, pp. 43–58.

Istance, D., Rees, G. and Williamson, H. (1994) *Young People not in Education, Training or Employment in South Glamorgan* Cardiff: South Glamorgan Training and Enterprise Council.

Jewson, N. and Mason, D. (1986) 'The Theory and Practice of EO Policies: liberal and radical approaches' *Sociological Review* Vol. 34, No. 2, pp. 591–617.

Jewson, N., Mason, D., Drewtt, A. and Rossiter, W. (1995) *Formal Equal Opportunities Policies and Employment Best Practice* Department for Education and Employment Research Series No. 69, London: DfEE.

Jones, H. C. (1996) 'The Contribution of the Structural Funds to Promoting Equal Opportunities', Paper delivered at the European Commission's conference *The European Union's Structural Funds and Equal Opportunities*, held in Brussels, 7–8 March 1996.

Kahn, P. (1992) 'Introduction: Equal Pay for Work of Equal Value in Britain and the USA' in P. Kahn and E. Meehan (eds) *Equal Value/Equal Worth in the UK and USA* Basingstoke: Macmillan.

Kahn, P. and Meehan, E. (eds) (1992) *Equal Value/Equal Worth in the UK and USA* Basingstoke: Macmillan.

Kandola, R. and Fullerton, J. (1994) *Managing the Mosaic – Diversity in Action* London: Institute of Personnel and Development.

Kanter, R. (1976) *Men and Women of the Corporation* New York: Basic Books.

Kennedy, M., Lubelska, C. and Walsh, V. (eds) (1993) *Making Connections: Women's Studies, Women's Movements, Women's Lives* London: Taylor and Francis.

Kirkup, G. and von Prümmer, C. (1997) 'Distance Education for European Women: The Threats and Opportunities of New Educational Forms and Media' *European Journal of Women's Studies*, Vol. 4, No. 2, pp. 39–62.

Lampard, R. (1994) 'Comment on Blackburn, Jarman and Siltanen: Marginal Matching and the Gini Coefficient' *Work, Employment and Society* Vol. 8, No. 3, pp. 407–12.

Lane, C. (1988) 'New Technology and Clerical Work' in D. Gallie (ed.) *Employment in Britain* Oxford: Blackwell.

Langkau-Herrmann, M. (1990) *In-company Vocational Training Programmes of Messerschmitt-Bolkow-Blohm GmbH (MBB)* Berlin: CEDEFOP.

Lawrence, E. (1994) *Gender and Trade Unions* London: Taylor and Francis.

Le Grand, J. and Bartlett, W. (eds) (1993) *Quasi Markets and Social Policy* London: Macmillan.

Lefebvre, M-C. (1993) *Evaluation of Women's Involvement in European Social Fund Co-financed Measures in 1990: Final Report for DGV, Social Europe Supplement 2/93* Luxembourg: Office for Official Publications of the European Communities.

Leonard, A. (1987a) *Judging Inequality: the effectiveness of the tribunal system in Sex Discrimination and Equal Pay cases* London: Cobden Trust.

—— (1987b) *Pyrrhic Victories: Winning Sex Discrimination and Equal Pay Cases in the Industrial Tribunals 1980–84* London: HMSO.

Levitas, R. (1996) 'The Concept of Social Exclusion and the new Durkheimian Hegemony' *Critical Social Policy* Vol. 16, No. 1, pp. 5–20.

Liff, S. (1996) *Managing Diversity: New Opportunities for Women* Warwick Papers in Industrial Relations No. 57, Warwick: University of Warwick School of Industrial and Business Studies Industrial Relations Research Unit.

Logue, H. A. and Talapessy, L. M. (eds) (1993) *Women in Science: International Workshop Proceedings* Brussels: DGXII, Commission of the European Communities.

Lovering, J. (1990) 'A Perfunctory sort of Post-Fordism: economic restructuring and labour market segmentation in Britain in the 1990s' *Work Employment and Society: The 1980s: A Decade of Change?* Special Issue, May, pp. 9–28.

MacEwan Scott, A. (ed.) (1994) *Gender Segregation and Social Change* Oxford: Oxford University Press.

McAdam, J. (1994) *Women in Contract Cleaning, Dublin* Report of the NOW steering committee, Dublin.

McGiveney, V. (1994) *Wasted Potential: Training and Career Progression for Part-time and Temporary Workers* Leicester: NIACE (National Organisation for Adult Learning).

McRae, S. (1996) *Women at the Top: progress after five years. A follow up report to the Hansard Society Commission on Women at the Top*, King Hall Paper No. 2, London: Hansard Society.

Maier, F. (1995) 'Wage and Non-Wage Labour Costs, Social Security and Public Funds to Combat Unemployment' in European Commission *Equal Opportunities for Women and Men: Follow-up to the White Paper on Growth, Competitiveness and Employment* Report to the European Commission's Task Force (Directorate-General V) Brussels: DGV European Commission V/5538/95-EN.

Maiworm, F., Steube, W. and Teichler, U. (1992) *Experiences of ERASMUS Students 1990/91* Kassel: Wissenschaftlichtes Zentrum für Berufs- und Hochschulforschung an der Gesamthochschule Kassel.

Marsh, C. (1988) 'Unemployment in Britain' in D. Gallie (ed.) *Employment in Britain* Oxford: Blackwell.

Marshall, J. (1995) *Women Managers Moving On: Exploring Career and Life Choices* London: Routledge.

Martin, J. and Roberts, C. (1984) *The Women and Employment Survey: A Lifetime Perspective*, London: HMSO.

Maruani, M. (1995) 'Inequalities and Flexibility' in European Commission *Equal Opportunities for Women and Men: Follow-up to the White Paper on Growth, Competitiveness and Employment* Report to the European Commission's Task Force (Directorate-General V) Brussels: DGV European Commission V/5538/95-EN.

Massey, D. (1993) 'Scientists, Transcendence, and the Work/Home Boundary' in J. Wajcman (ed.) *Organisations, Gender and Power* Warwick Papers in Industrial Relations No. 8, Coventry: Industrial Relations Research Unit, University of Warwick .

Maurice, M., Sellier, F. and Silvestre, J-J. (1986) *The Social Foundations of Industrial Power* London: MIT Press.

May, A. (1987) *Equal Opportunities and Vocational Training, Establishment and Management of Businesses by Women: a synthesis of twelve national reports and four complementary reports* Berlin: CEDEFOP.

Maynard, M. (1994) ' "Race" Gender and the Concept of Difference' in H. Afshar and M. Maynard (eds) *The Dynamics of 'Race' and Gender: Some Feminist Interventions* London: Taylor and Francis.

Mazey, S. (1988) 'European Community Action on behalf of women: the limits of legislation' *Journal of Common Market Studies* Vol. XXVII, pp. 63–84.

Meager, N. and Williams, M. (1994) *The Case for National 'Equality in Employment Targets'* A consultation paper prepared for the TEC National Council, Falmer: University of Sussex.

Meehan, E. (1993) *Citizenship and the European Community* London: Sage.

Meulders, D. (1995) 'Reorganisation of Work' in European Commission *Equal Opportunities for Women and Men: Follow-up to the White Paper on Growth, Competitiveness and Employment* Report to the European Commission's Task Force (Directorate-General V) Brussels: DGV European Commission V/5538/95-EN.

Meulders, D., Plasman, G. and Plasman, R. (1994) *Atypical Employment in the EC* Aldershot: Dartmouth Publishing.

Mitchell, M. and Russell, D. (1994) 'Race, citizenship and "Fortress Europe" ' in P. Brown and R. Crompton (eds) *Economic Restructuring and Social Exclusion* London: UCL Press.

Mitchell, S. (1984) *Tall Poppies: Successful Australian Women Talk to Susan Mitchell* Victoria: Penguin.

Mitter, S. (1986) *Common Fate, Common Bond: Women in the Global Economy* London: Pluto Press.

Morphy, L., Bynner, J. and Parsons, S. (1997) 'Gendered Skill Development' in H. Metcalf (ed.) *Half Our Future: Women, Skill Development and Training* London: Policy Studies Institute (in press).

Morris, L. (1990) *The Workings of the Household: A US UK Comparison* Oxford: Polity.

Moss, P. (1990a) 'Childcare in the European Communities 1985–90' *Women of Europe Supplement*, No. 31, Brussels: Commission of the European Communities.

—— (1990b) 'Childcare and equality of opportunity' in M. O'Brien, L. Hantrais and S. Mangeen (eds) *Women, Equal Opportunities and Welfare* Aston University Cross National Research Papers, New Series, The Implications of 1992 for Social Policy, Birmingham: Aston University.

Muir, E. J. (1994a) *Enterprising Women in Europe: Education, Training, Personal and Business Support* Brussels: European Commission, DGV Equal Opportunities Unit.

—— (1994b) 'Enterprising Women in Europe: Balancing Private and Public Lives' *Equal Opportunities International*, Vol. 13, Nos 3/4/5, pp. 39–49.

—— (1997) *Enterprising Women in Europe* Unpublished PhD thesis, University of Bristol.

Mungham, G. (1982) 'Workless Youth as a "Moral Panic" ' in T. Rees and

P. Atkinson (eds) *Youth Unemployment and State Intervention* London: Routledge and Kegan Paul.

National Advisory Council for Education and Training Targets (1994) *Report on Progress* London: NACETT Department of Employment.

Neave, G. (1990) 'Policy and Response: Changing Perceptions and Priorities in the Vocational Training Policy of the EEC' in G. Esland (ed.) *Education, Training and Employment: Vol. 2, The Educational Response* Wokingham: Addison-Wesley in association with the Open University.

Newton, P. (1991) 'Computing: an ideal occupation for women?' in J. Firth-Cozens and M. West (eds) *Women at Work* Milton Keynes: Open University Press.

NIACE (1996) *Adults Learning. Special Issue: Women and the European Year of Lifelong Learning* Vol. 8, No. 2, Leicester: NIACE.

Nicholl, W. and Salmon, T. C. (1994) *Understanding the New European Communities* 2nd edn, Hemel Hempstead: Harvester Wheatsheaf.

Nielson, R. and Szyszczak, E. (1991) *The Social Dimension of the European Community* Copenhagen: Handelshojskolens Forlag.

Nugent, N. (1994) *The Government and Politics of the European Union* 3rd edn, Basingstoke: Macmillan.

O'Brien, A. (1992) 'Participation of Women in the COMETT Programme', Documents 1, 2 and 3 prepared for TFHR, Brussels: COMETT Technical Assistance Office.

O'Donovan, K. and Szyszczak, E. (1988) *Equality and Sex Discrimination Law* Oxford: Blackwell.

OECD (1986) *New Information Technologies: a challenge for education* Paris: OECD.

—— (1994) *Women and Structural Change: New Perspectives* Paris: OECD.

PA Cambridge Economic Consultants (1992) *An Evaluation of the IRIS Network* Cambridge: PA Cambridge Economic Consultants.

Pahl, R. E. (1984) *Divisions of Labour* Oxford: Blackwell.

Payne, J. (1994) *Responses to qualifications: a comparison of paths after compulsory schooling* ED Research Series, Youth Cohort Report, London: Employment Department.

Peck, J. A. (1991) 'Letting the market decide (with public money): Training and Enterprise Councils and the future of labour market programmes' *Critical Social Policy* Vol. 31, No. 4, pp. 4–17.

Pelgrum, W. J. and Plomp, T. (1991) *The Use of Computers in Education Worldwide* Oxford: Pergamon Press/International Association for the Evaluation of Educational Achievement.

PETRA Technical Assistance Office (1989) *Survey of the number and characteristics of the beneficiaries of PETRA YIPs* Brussels: PETRA TAO.

—— (1991) *ENTP Survey* Brussels: PETRA TAO.

Phillips, A. (1987) *Feminism and Equality* Oxford: Basil Blackwell.

Phillips, A. and Taylor, B. (1980) 'Sex and Skill: Notes towards a feminist economics' *Feminist Review* No. 6, pp. 79–88.

Phizacklea, A. and Wolkowitz, C. (1995) *Homeworking Women: Gender, Racism and Class at Work* London: Sage.

Pilcher J., Delamont, S., Powell, G. and Rees, T. (1988) 'Women's Training Roadshows and the "manipulation" of schoolgirls' career choices' *British Journal of Education and Work* Vol. 2, No. 2, pp. 61–6.

Pillinger, J. (1992) *Feminising the Market: Women's Pay and Employment in the European Community* Basingstoke: Macmillan.

Plantenga, J. and Tijdens, K. (1995) 'Segregation in the European Union: Developments in the 1980s' in A. van Doorne-Huiskes, J. van Hoof and E. Roelofs (eds) *Women and the European Labour Markets* London: Paul Chapman Publishing.

Pollert, A. and Rees, T. (1992) 'Equal Opportunity and Positive Action in Britain: Three Case Studies' *Warwick Papers in Industrial Relations No. 42* Coventry: University of Warwick Industrial Relations Research Unit, School of Industrial and Business Studies.

Prechal, S. and Senden, L. (1994) *Monitoring Implementation and Application of Community Equality Law 1992–1993* Brussels: DGV European Commission.

Prechal, S., Senden, L. and van der Meij, H. (1994) *Law Network Newsletter 2* Summer 1994, Brussels: DGV European Commission.

Pugliese, E. (1995) 'Youth Unemployment and the Condition of Young Women in the Labour Market' in European Commission *Equal Opportunities for Women and Men: Follow-up to the White Paper on Growth, Competitiveness and Employment* Report to the European Commission's Task Force (Directorate-General V) Brussels: DGV European Commission V/5538/95-EN.

Rainbird, H. (1993) 'Vocational education and training' in M. Gold (ed.) *The Social Dimension: Employment Policy in the European Community* London: Macmillan.

Ramazanoglu, C. (1987) 'Sex and Violence in Academic Life or You Can Keep a Good Woman Down' in J. Hanmer and M. Maynard (eds) *Women, Violence and Social Control* London: Macmillan.

—— (1989) 'Improving on Sociology: Problems in taking a feminist standpoint' *Sociology*, Vol. 23, No. 3, pp. 427–45.

Rees, C. and Willox, I. (1991) *Expanding the role of women in the South Wales Labour Force* Cardiff: Welsh Development Agency.

Rees, G. (1990) *New Information Technologies and Vocational Education and Training in the European Community: The Challenge of the 1990s* Report to the Task Force Human Resources, Education, Training and Youth, Employment and Training Perspectives in the New Information Technologies in the European Community Project, Cardiff: School of Social and Administrative Studies, University of Wales Cardiff.

Rees, G. and Fielder, S. (1992) 'The Services Economy, Subcontracting and New Employment Relations: contract catering and cleaning' *Work, Employment and Society* Vol. 6, No. 3, pp. 347–65.

Rees, G., Fielder, S. and Rees, T. (1992) *Employees' Access to Training Opportunities; Shaping the Social Structure of Labour Markets* Cardiff: School of Social and Administrative Studies, University of Wales Cardiff.

Rees, G., Rees, T. and Fielder, S. (1991) *Training Needs and Provision: The Bridgend Case Study* Institutional Determinants of Adult Training, End of Award Report to ESRC (Grant No. XC1125009) Cardiff: School of Social and Administrative Studies, University of Wales Cardiff.

Rees, G., Williamson, H. and Istance, D. (1996) ' "Status Zero": Jobless School-leavers in South Wales' *Research Papers in Education* Vol. 11, pp. 219–35.

Rees, T. (1980) *Study of Schemes of Direct Job Creation in Northern Ireland* Brussels: DGV, Commission of the European Communities.

—— (1983) 'Boys off the Street and Girls in the Home: Youth Unemployment and State Intervention in Northern Ireland' in R. Fiddy (ed.) *In Place of Work: Policy and Provision for the Young Unemployed* Lewes: Falmer.

—— (1992a) *Skill Shortages, Women and the New Information Technologies* Luxembourg: Office for Official Publications of the European Communities.

—— (1992b) *Women and the Labour Market* London: Routledge.

—— (1994a) 'Feminising the Mainstream: Women and the European Union's Training Policies' *Equal Opportunities International*, Vol. 13, Nos 3/4/5, pp. 9–28.

—— (1994b) 'Information Technology Skills and Access to Training Opportunities: Germany and the UK' in K. Ducatel (ed.) *Employment and Technical Change in Europe: Work Organization, Skills and Training* Aldershot: Edward Elgar.

—— (1994c) 'Women and Paid Work in Wales' in J. Aaron, T. Rees, S. Betts and M. Vincentelli (eds) *Our Sisters' Land: The Changing Identities of Women in Wales* Cardiff: University of Wales Press.

—— (1994d) *Women employees' training needs in Wales, Catalonia, Dublin and Thessaloniki* An EC FORCE Project, Cardiff: Welsh Development Agency.

—— (1995a) 'Equality into Education and Training Policies' in European Commission *Equal Opportunities for Women and Men: Follow-up to the White Paper on Growth, Competitiveness and Employment* Report to the European Commission's Task Force (Directorate-General V) Brussels: DGV European Commission V/5538/95-EN.

—— (1995b) *Women and the EC Training Programmes: Tinkering, Tailoring, Transforming* Bristol: University of Bristol, SAUS Publications.

—— (1995c) 'Women and Training Policy in the EU' *Gender, Work and Organization* Vol. 2, No. 1, pp. 34–45.

Rees, T., Doogan, K., Redmond, D. and Stokes, P. (1980) *Study of Schemes of Direct Job Creation in the Republic of Ireland* Brussels: DGV, Commission of the European Communities.

Rees, T. and Fielder, S. (1992) 'Through the Dark Glass Ceiling: Women and Top Jobs in Wales' *Contemporary Wales* Vol. 5, Cardiff: University of Wales Press, pp. 99–114.

Rees, T., Heaton, P. and McBriar, L. (1998) 'Women in Education in Northern Ireland' in S. Riddell and J. Salisbury (eds) *Gender Equality Policies and Educational Reforms in the UK* Lewes: Falmer Press (in press).

Rees, T. and Varlaam, C. (1983) *The Experience of Girls in the EC Pilot*

Projects on the Transition from School to Working Life Cologne: IFAPLAN.

Reskin, B. and Hartmann, H. (eds) (1986) *Women's Work, Men's Work: Sex Segregation on the Job* Washington DC: National Academy Press.

Robbins, D. *et al.* (1994) *National policies to combat social exclusion* (Third Annual Report of the European Observatory on Policies to Combat Social Exclusion) Brussels: European Commission.

Roelofs, S. (1995) 'The European Equal Opportunities Policy' in A. van Doorne-Huiskes, J. van Hoof and E. Roelofs (eds) *Women and the European Labour Markets* Heerlen: Open University and Paul Chapman Publishing.

Room, G. (ed.) (1995) *Beyond the Threshold: the Measurement and Analysis of Social Exclusion* Bristol: Policy Press.

Ross, R. and Schneider, R. (1992) *From Equality to Diversity* London: Pitman.

Rossilli, M. (1997) 'The European Community's Policy on the Equality of Women: From the Treaty of Rome to the present' *European Journal of Women's Studies*, Vol. 4, No. 1, pp. 63–82.

Routledge, P. (1996) *Madam Speaker: A Biography* London: HarperCollins.

Rubery, J. and Fagan, C. (1993) *Occupational Segregation amongst Women and Men in the European Community* Social Europe 393, Luxembourg: Office for Official Publications of the European Communities.

Rubery, J. and Fagan, C. with Grimshaw, D. (1994) *Wage Determination and Sex Segregation in Employment in the European Community* Social Europe Supplement 4/94, Luxembourg: Office for Official Publications of the European Communities.

Rubery, J., Fagan, C. and Humphries, J. (1992) *Occupational Segregation in the UK* Report for DGV, European Commission Network on the Situation of Women in the Labour Market, Brussels: European Commission.

Rubery, J. and Humphries, J. (eds) (1995) *The Economics of Equal Opportunities* Manchester: Equal Opportunities Commission.

Rubery, J., Smith, M. and Fagan, P. (1995) *Occupational Segregation of Men and Women and Atypical Work in the European Union* Brussels: DGV, European Commission (V/5619/95-EN).

Salisbury, J. (1996) *Educational Reforms and Gender Inequality in Welsh Schools* Manchester: Equal Opportunities Commission.

Sargeant, G. (1989) *Returners' Research Project: A Report for the Training Agency on Women into the Labour Market* Hatfield Heath, Herts: Dow Stoker.

Schiersmann, C. (ed.) (1988) *Mehr Risiken als Chancen? Frauen und Neue Technologien* Hanover: Institut Frau und Gesellschaft.

Schwartz, B. (1981) *The Integration of Young People in Society and Working Life* Report by Bertrand Schwartz for the Prime Minister of France, Berlin: CEDEFOP.

Senker, J. and Senker, P. (1994a) 'Core IT Skills and Employment' in K. Ducatel (ed.) *Employment and Technical Change in Europe: Work Organization, Skills and Training* Aldershot: Edward Elgar.

—— (1994b) 'Information Technology and Skills in Manufacturing and

Construction' K. Ducatel (ed.) *Employment and Technical Change in Europe: Work Organization, Skills and Training* Aldershot: Edward Elgar.

Senker, P. and Senker, J. (1994c) 'Skills Implications of Technical Change in the Service Sector' in K. Ducatel (ed.) *Employment and Technical Change in Europe: Work Organization, Skills and Training* Aldershot: Edward Elgar.

Serdjenian, E. (1994) 'Inventory of Positive Action in Europe' *Women of Europe Supplement*, No. 42, Brussels: Commission of the European Communities.

Seward-Thompson, B. (1987) 'Attitudes in the IT Industry – the key to the future' *Information Technology and Public Policy* Vol. 6, pp. 25–7.

Siltanen, J., Jarman, J. and Blackburn, R. M. (1994) *Gender Inequality in the Labour Market: Occupational Concentration and Segregation, a Manual on Methodology* (rev. edn), Geneva: International Labour Organisation.

Skinner, J. and Coyle, A. (1988) 'Women at Work in Social Services' in A. Coyle and J. Skinner (eds) *Women and Work: Positive Action for Change* London: Macmillan.

Sloane, P. J. (1994) 'The Gender Wage Differential and Discrimination in the six SCELI Local Labour Markets' in A. MacEwan Scott (ed.) *Gender Segregation and Social Change* Oxford: Oxford University Press (The Social Change and Economic Life Initiative).

Smith, D. (1987) *The Everyday World as Problematic: a feminist sociology* Milton Keynes: Open University Press.

Smith, J. (1993a) *Athena: Women Entrepreneurs, Skills Training and Enterprise Development* Cardiff: Welsh Development Agency, Report to The European Commission Task Force Human Resources, Education, Training and Youth.

—— (1993b) *Athena Synthesis Report* Cardiff: Welsh Development Agency, Report to The European Commission Task Force Human Resources, Education, Training and Youth.

Snape, D., Thomson, K. and Chetwynd, M. (1995) *Discrimination against Gay Men and Lesbians* London: Social and Community Planning Research.

Spencer, A. and Podmore, D. (1987) *In a Man's World: Essays on Women in Male Dominated Professions* London: Tavistock.

Spencer, L. and Taylor, S. (1994) 'Participation and Progress in the Labour Market: key issues for women' *Research Series* No. 35, London: Employment Department .

Spender, D. (1995) *Nattering on the Net: Women, Power and Cyberspace* Melbourne: Spinifex.

Squires, J. (1994) 'Beyond the liberal conception of equal opportunity', Paper delivered to the Equity, Labour and Social Divisions Initiative, Faculty of Social Sciences, University of Bristol (mimeo).

Stolte-Heiskanen, V. and Furst-Dilic, R. (1991) *Women in Science, Token Women or Gender Equality?* Oxford/New York: Berg.

Sullerot, E. (1991) *A Practical Manual on how to create and run positive action training programmes for women only, how to create and run positive action programmes to promote women inside companies* Brussels: Commission of the European Communities, Directorate General Employment, Industrial Relations and Social Affairs.

Swann, Lord (1985) *The Report of the Committee of Inquiry into the Education of Children from Ethnic Minority Groups* Cmnd 9453, London: HMSO.

Taking Liberties Collective (1989) *Learning the Hard Way: Women's Oppression in Men's Education* London: Macmillan.

Tannen, D. (1995) *Talking From Nine to Five – Women and Men at Work: Language, Sex and Power* London: Virago.

Tanton, M. (ed.) (1994) *Women in Management: a developing presence* London: Routledge.

Task Force Human Resources, Education, Training and Youth (1990) *Equal Opportunities and New Information Technologies* Brussels: Commission of the European Communities.

—— (1991) *The Added Value of Community Measures Relating to the Introduction of New Information Technology in Education* (draft communication), Brussels: Commission of the European Communities.

—— (1992) *TEMPUS Trans-European Mobility Scheme for University Students: Annual Report 7 May 1990/31 July 1991* Brussels: Commission of the European Communities.

Teichler, U. (1991) *Experiences of ERASMUS Students: Select Findings of the 1988/90 Survey* Kassel: Wissenschaftlichtes Zentrum für Berufs- und Hochschulforschung an der Gesamthochschule Kassel.

Teichler, U., Kreitz, R. and Maiworm, F. (1990) *Student Mobility within ERASMUS 1987/88: A Statistical Survey* Kassel: Wissenschaftlichtes Zentrum für Berufs- und Hochschulforschung an der Gesamthochschule Kassel.

—— (1991a) *Student Mobility within ERASMUS 1988/89: A Statistical Profile* Kassel: Wissenschaftlichtes Zentrum für Berufs- und Hochschulforschung an der Gesamthochschule Kassel.

—— (1991b) *Student Mobility within ERASMUS 1989/90: A Statistical Profile* Kassel: Wissenschaftlichtes Zentrum für Berufs- und Hochschulforschung an der Gesamthochschule Kassel.

—— (1992) *Student Mobility within ERASMUS 1990/91: A Statistical Profile* Kassel: Wissenschaftlichtes Zentrum für Berufs- und Hochschulforschung an der Gesamthochschule Kassel.

Tierney, M. (1995) 'Negotiating a Software Career: informal work practices and "The lads" in a software installation' in K. Grint and R. Gill (eds) *The Gender-Technology Relations: Contemporary Theory and Research* London: Taylor and Francis.

Tijdens, K. (1991) 'Decentralised office technology and women's work' in P. van den Bessalar, A. Clement and P. Jarvinnen (eds) *Information System, Work and Organization Design* Amsterdam: North-Holland.

Townsend, P. (1979) *Poverty in the United Kingdom* Harmondsworth: Penguin.

Trades Union Congress (1989) *Skills 2000* London: TUC.

Training and Employment Agency (1996) *'Status O': A Socio-economic*

Study of Young People on the Margin Belfast: Training and Employment Agency.

van Doorne-Huiskes, A., van Hoof, J. and Roelefs, E. (eds) (1995) *Women and the European Labour Markets* Heerlen: Open University/Paul Chapman Publishing.

van Overbeek, J. P. M. (1994) *Handbook on Equal Treatment between Men and Women in the European Community* Brussels: European Commission, DGV V/A/3, Equal Opportunities Unit.

Vickery, K. (1990) *Impact of the Current Economic Climate on IT* London: PA Consulting Group.

Violi, P. (1992) 'Gender, subjectivity and language' in G. Bock and S. James (eds) *Beyond Equality and Difference* London: Routledge.

Virgo, P. (1991) 'The Key to Overcoming Your IT Skills Problems: The Case for Joining the Women into IT Foundation' Farnborough: Women into IT Foundation Ltd (mimeo).

Von Prondzynski, F. (1986) *Implementation of the Equality Directives* Luxembourg: Office for Official Publications of the European Union.

Wajcman, J. (1991) *Feminism Confronts Technology* Oxford: Polity.

Walby, S. (ed.) (1988) *Gender Segregation at Work* Milton Keynes: Open University Press.

—— (1990) *Theorising Patriarchy* Oxford: Blackwell.

—— (1994/95) 'Gender, Work and Post-Fordism: The EC Context' in *International Journal of Sociology* Vol. 24, No. 4, pp. 67–82.

Warde, A. and Hetherington, K. (1993) 'A Changing Domestic Division of Labour? Issues of Measurement and Interpretation' *Work, Employment and Society* Vol. 7, No. 1, pp. 23–45.

Warner, H. (1984) 'EC Social Policy in Practice: community action on behalf of women and its impact in the member states' *Journal of Common Market Studies* Vol. XXIII, pp. 141–67.

Watson, S. (1989) *Winning Women: The Price of Success in a Man's World* London: Weidenfeld and Nicolson.

Watts, M. J. (1994) 'A Critique of Marginal Matching' *Work, Employment and Society* Vol. 8, No. 3, pp. 421–32.

Webb, J. and Liff, S. (1988) 'Play the White Man: the social construction of fairness and competition in equal opportunities policies' *Sociological Review* Vol. 36, No. 3, pp. 532–51.

Weber, M. (1968) *Economy and Society* (ed. G. Roth and C. Wittich) New York: Bedminster Press.

Webster, J. (1996) *Shaping Women's Work: Gender, Employment and Information Technology* London: Longman.

Weedon, C. (1987) *Feminist Practice and Post Structuralist Theory* Oxford: Blackwell.

Wellington, J. J. (1989) *Education for Employment: The Place of Information Technology* Windsor: National Foundation for Education Research.

Welsh, C., Knox, J. and Brett, M. (1994) *Acting Positively: Positive Action Under the Race Relations Act 1976* Sheffield: Employment Department.

Welsh Office (1995) *People and Prosperity: An Agenda for Action in Wales* Cardiff: Welsh Office.

Wenger, C. (1995) 'Old Women in Rural Wales' in J. Aaron, T. Rees, S. Betts and M. Vincentelli (eds) *Our Sisters' Land: the changing identities of women in Wales* Cardiff: University of Wales Press.

West, J. and Lyon, K. (1995) 'The Trouble with Equal Opportunities: the case of women academics' *Gender and Education* Vol. 7, No. 1, pp. 51–68.

Whitting, G. and Quinn, J. (1989) 'Women and work: preparing for an independent future' *Policy and Politics* Vol. 17, No. 4, pp. 337–46.

Whyte, J., Deem, R., Cant, L. and Cruickshank, M. (eds) (1985) *Girl-Friendly Schooling* London: Methuen.

Wilkinson, C. (1995) *The Drop Out Society: Young People on the Margin* Leicester: Youth Work Press.

Willis, L. and Daisley, J. (1990) *Springboard Women's Development Workshop* Stroud: Hawthorn Press.

Wilpert, C. (ed.) (1996) *Zukunftsausseichetn-Chancengleichheit in der beruflichen Bildung von Frauen in Europa* Abschlusstagung der nationalen koordinierungstelle des IRIS-Netzwerks in Deutschland, Dezember 1995, in Berlin, Berlin: Bundesinstitut für Berufsbildung.

Witherspoon, S. (1988) 'Interim Report: A Woman's Work' in R. Jowell, S. Witherspoon and L. Brook (eds) *British Social Attitudes: The 5th Report, 1988/89 Edition* Aldershot: Gower/Social and Community Planning Research.

Wollstonecraft, M. (1967 [1792]) *The Vindication of the Rights of Woman* New York: W. W. Norton & Co.

Women's National Commission, Equal Opportunities Commission and Equal Opportunities Commission for Northern Ireland (1996) *In Pursuit of Equality: National Agenda for Action Policy Papers* London: Women's National Commission.

Woodfield, R. (1994) *An ethnographic exploration of some factors which mediate between gender and skill in a software R&D unit* Unpublished PhD thesis, University of Sussex, Science Policy Research Unit.

Wrench, J. and Solomos, J. (1995) *Racism and Migration in Western Europe* Oxford: Berg.

Wulf-Matheis, M. (1997) 'The Structural Funds and Equal Opportunities' in Chwarae Teg (Fair Play) (eds) *Women, Players in Regional Development* Cardiff: Chwarae Teg.

Young, I. M. (1990) *Justice and the Politics of Difference* Princeton NJ: Princeton University Press.

Index

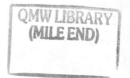